Celebrating
NURSES
A VISUAL HISTORY

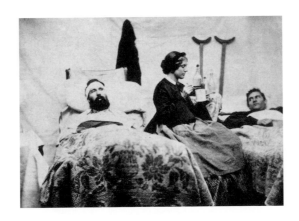

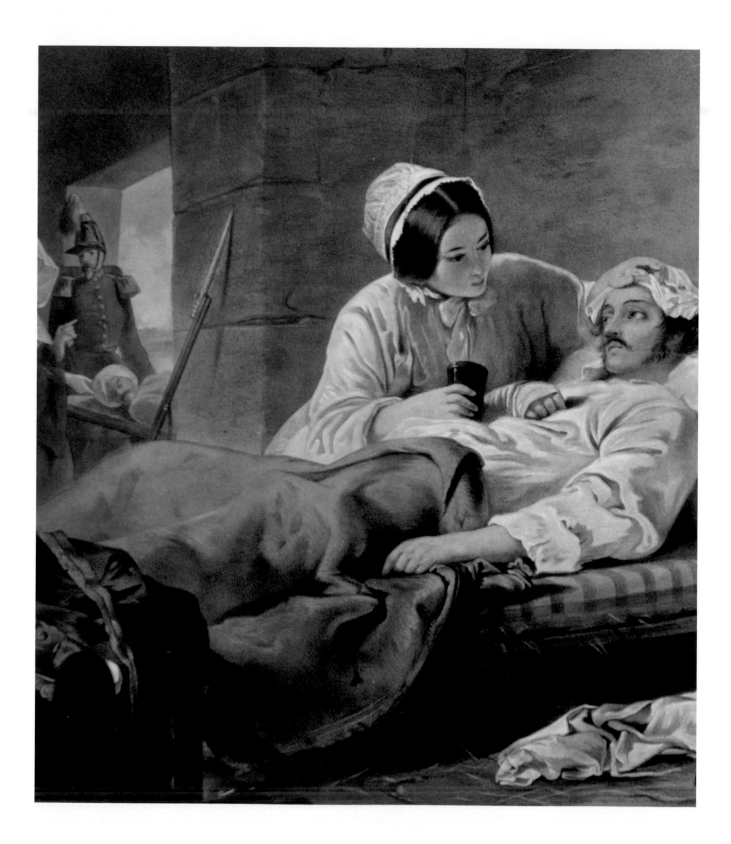

Celebrating NURSES
A VISUAL HISTORY

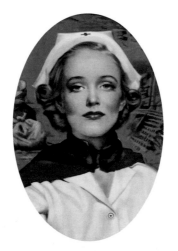

CHRISTINE E. HALLETT
FOREWORD BY JOAN E LYNAUGH, RN, MSN, PHD, FAAN

BARRON'S

To Margaret D. Hallett

Conceived, edited, and designed by Fil Rouge Press Ltd., 538 Ben Jonson House, Barbican, London EC2Y 8NH

First edition published in 2010 in the United States and Canada by Barron's Educational Series, Inc.
First published in the United Kingdom in 2010 by
Fil Rouge Press, 538 Ben Jonson House, London EC2Y 8NH

All inquiries should be addressed to:
Barron's Educational Series, Inc.
250 Wireless Boulevard
Hauppauge, New York 11788
www.barronseduc.com

ISBN-13: 978-0-7641-6286-2
ISBN-10: 0-7641-6286-1

Library of Congress Catalog Card No. 2009936586

Printed in Thailand by Imago

10 9 8 7 6 5 4 3 2 1

Publisher: Judith More
Editor: Miren Lopategui
Designer: Dave Jones
Picture Researcher: Emily Hedges

Contents

Foreword

Readers everywhere will enjoy and benefit from this sophisticated and beautifully illustrated history of nursing and caregiving since the beginning of recorded human history. Christine Hallett's amazing overview of nurses and nursing is an invaluable resource for all who are concerned about the future of health care. Here we rediscover how ubiquitous and essential nursing is to civil society everywhere. For more than one hundred and fifty years modern nursing has spread around the world, disregarding national boundaries and changing the experience of sickness and dependence. But Dr Hallett reminds us how much today's societies owe to our predecessors going back to ancient times. She reveals nursing in its fullest context and helps us examine what did happen and what is happening in nursing and health care in our world today. She also helps us see how beliefs about health, religions, science and gender helped shape the course of change. Moreover, she offers us context so that we can understand how rising expectations placed on nurses by the public accentuated investment in nursing as the twentieth century drew to a close. This is a book that skillfully employs major themes and personal stories to bring the history of nursing to life.

Finally, this book is an outstanding contribution to a still small but growing contemporary historiography of nursing. It is a significant achievement in international historical scholarship.

Joan E. Lynaugh

Right:
Front cover of a book by nurse-author Honnor Morten.

HOW TO BECOME A NURSE

BY HONNOR MORTEN.

Introduction

The story of nursing is an extraordinary and often moving one. It is the story of a group of people who developed, protected, and handed down through hundreds of generations the art of nurturing, supporting, and empowering their fellow human beings. It is also the story of extraordinary individuals, who devoted their working lives to the wellbeing of others.

There were times when these "carers" thrived—when the societies in which they worked recognized their value and supported their efforts. There were others, though, in which nurses were undermined and vilified—sometimes even persecuted. Nursing survived these dark times. It also survived many periods of indifference, when its work was taken for granted.

As we move into the second decade of the twenty-first century, it seems as though our world may be leaving behind one such period of indifference, as it begins to free itself from the individualistic, alienating ideas of the late twentieth century and allows itself to be governed by a new philosophy. This shift was expressed recently by U.S. President Barack Obama, who wrote that "we have a stake in one another, and that which binds us together is greater than that which drives us apart." In writing these words, Obama was, perhaps unconsciously, echoing one of the most famous and extraordinary nurses of modern times, Mother Teresa, who suggested that the world's problems had arisen because "we all recognize a family that is too small."

Nurses draw their family circle large. The art of nursing is the "care of strangers." Its practitioners perform work that is beyond the capacity of informal caregivers—families and friends. As our world begins to change, it seems timely to tell the story of this extraordinary group, who have sustained, unbroken, a thread of knowledge, skill, and wisdom that holds our ability as human beings to care for and sustain each other. Nurses are, as Patricia Donahue said, among the greatest artists the world has ever known; yet the performance of their art takes place in secret, and the majority of us know little about it. As this book tells the story of nurses, it will dip into a rich vein of history, and, because it would be impossible to recount that history in its entirety, only small fragments will be told. Although the lives and works of some famous nurses will be portrayed, the book will also bring to light the hidden work of individuals who, though less well-known, were no less extraordinary.

Christine E. Hallett

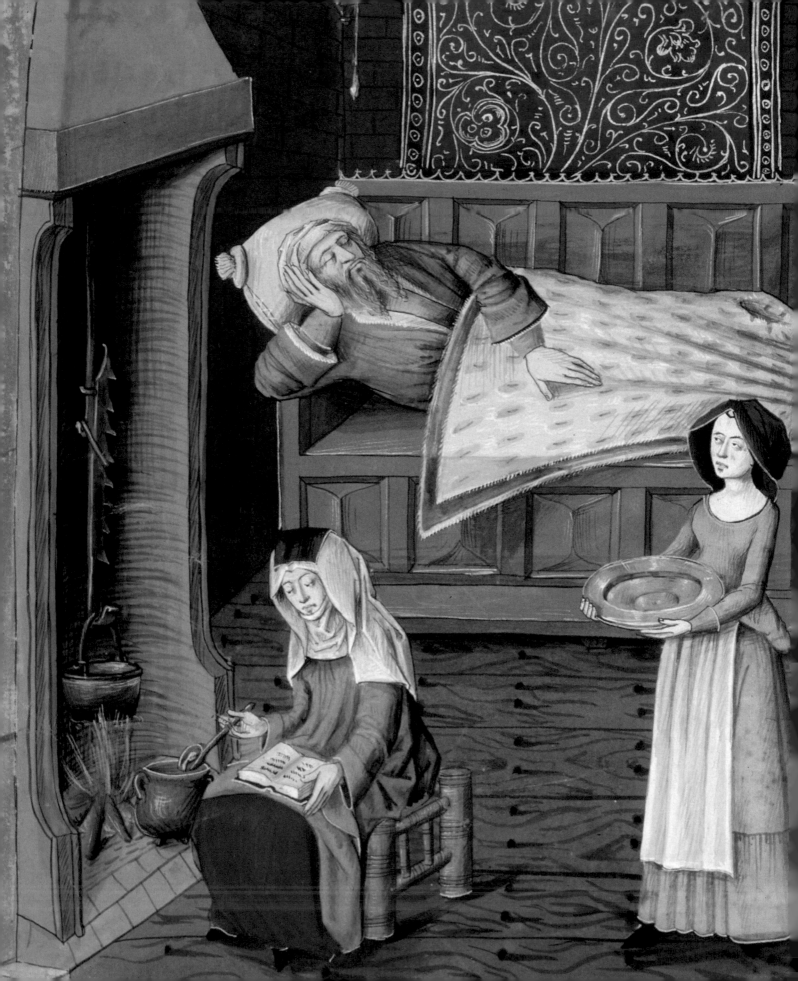

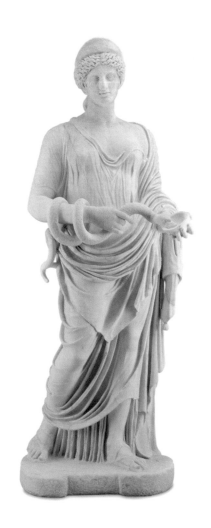

1 BEGINNINGS

Although nursing was not established as a professional discipline until the nineteenth century, the concept of caring for the sick has been with us since earliest times. The healing work of nurses developed and advanced from the earliest civilizations to the end of the eighteenth century.

Ancient Times

Human society has always recognized the need to care for the sick. Early societies had healers known as shamans, who held and passed on a detailed knowledge of the healing properties of plants, minerals, and crystals. These "witch doctors" were revered and respected, but were also often feared, because they drew their power from the widespread belief that illness was caused by evil spirits. Shamans can be seen as some of history's earliest nurses, but the concept of nursing was also well established among the women of these societies, who simply extended their natural role as carers of children and the elderly.

EARLY CIVILIZATIONS

The earliest known civilizations—those of the ancient Egyptians, Babylonians, and Assyrians—left written and visual records of their ideas about healing. But while it is clear that healing and medicine played a central role in these societies, the records say little about those who provided hands-on bedside care for the sick or who promoted the health of ordinary people. Only elite members of society, such as the famous Egyptian physician Imhotep, are mentioned. Such priest-physicians were believed to have sacred powers. They continued the tradition by which the earliest groups of human beings attributed magical or spiritual powers to those who could heal the sick.

CLASSICAL GREECE

In Ancient Greece, religion and healing were closely linked in the worship of Asklepios, the god of healing, who was said to cure the sick through dreams. From around 500 B.C., healing sanctuaries, or asklepions, dedicated to his worship were established all over the country. These centers were both temples and hospitals and the healing that took place in them was seen as a sacred and divine process. Patients entering the asklepion left the world behind and remained in sanctuary for several days or even weeks. The process of healing seems strange to modern eyes. After *Katharsis*, or purification, in a series of cleansing baths, patients fell into a trancelike sleep (often induced by hallucinogenic drugs) and then dreamed their own cures—which were promptly implemented. During these processes they were waited upon by attendants who cared for their needs, administered their medications, and offered them emotional and spiritual support. These attendants were said to be priests, but, like the shamans, they may be seen as some of history's earliest nurses.

Whatever you may feel about the administration of hallucinogenic drugs, the information we have on asklepions suggests that patients often emerged from them feeling better. These were clearly places of sanctuary where mental rest, sleep, and nutritious food were important parts of the cure.

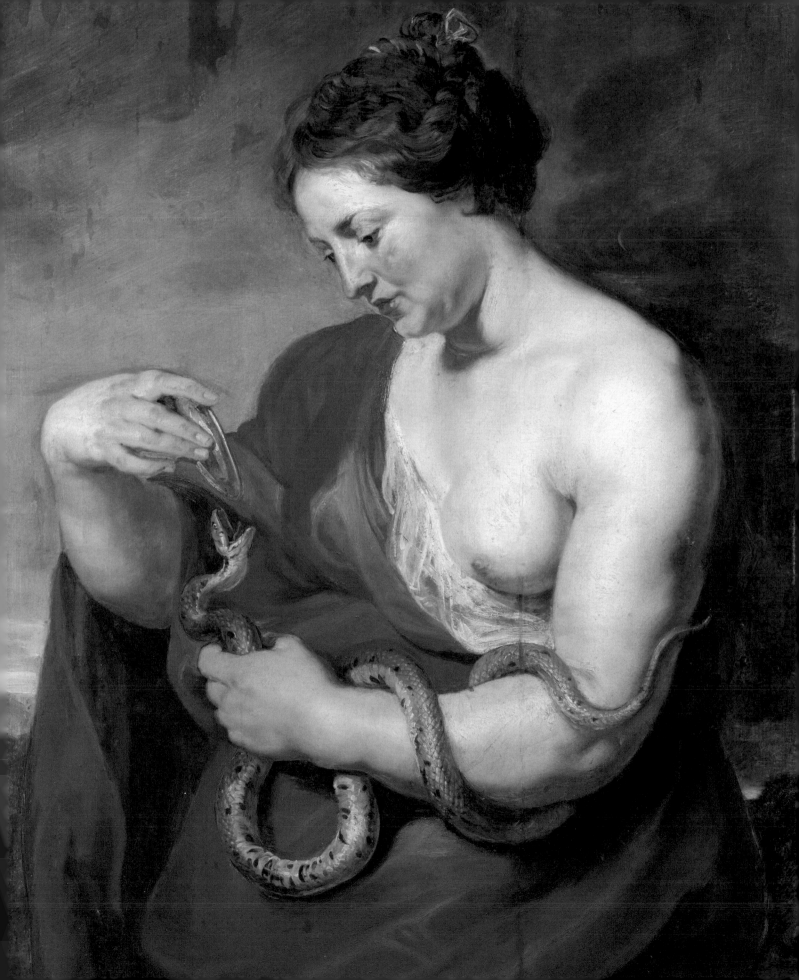

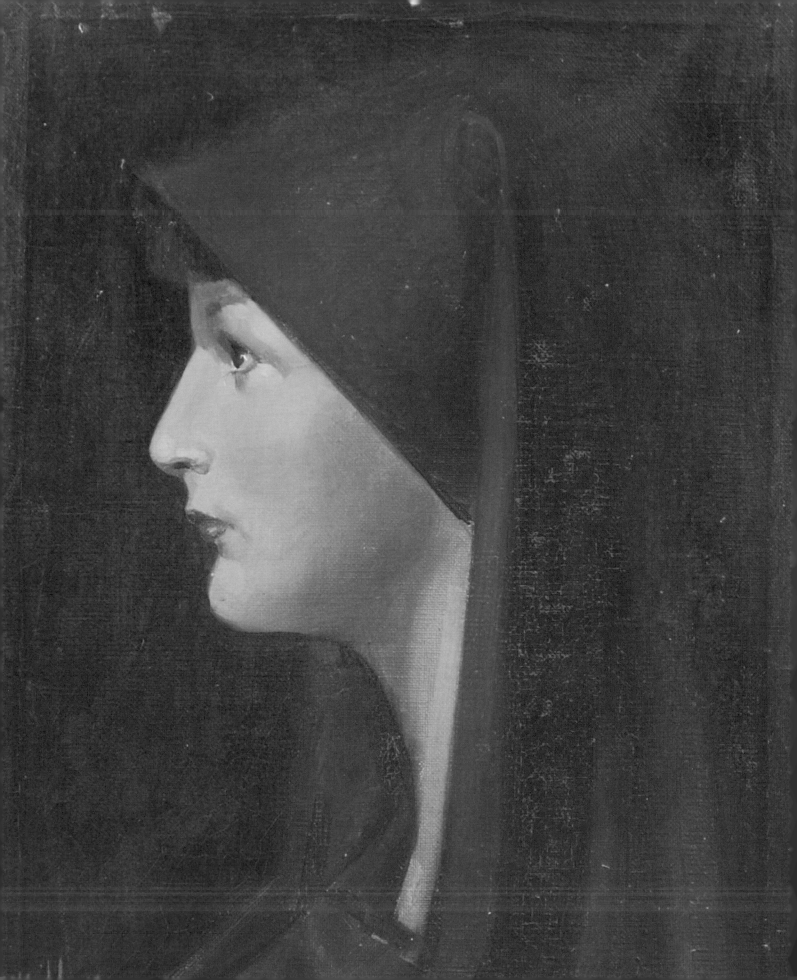

THE ROMAN EMPIRE

The records and writings of Ancient Rome are silent upon the subject of nursing, until the first century A.D., when Christianity was beginning to develop in the Roman Empire. The Christian religion has had a hugely important influence on the way in which nursing has developed, and is inextricably linked with the work of those early nurses who decided to dedicate themselves to the service of others.

The Christian emphasis on self-sacrifice—putting aside one's own worldly interests in order to serve others—meant that nursing the sick became a highly valued pursuit. It was also highly dangerous in a time when infectious diseases, for which there was no known cure, were rife. The sicker the patient (and therefore the more dangerous the work), the more likely were the individual's actions to be valued by a God who could see and understand everything. The higher goal for those who nursed the sick (apart from the obvious satisfaction of saving lives) was their own "salvation," a reward obtained after death in another spiritual dimension—a "heaven" or "paradise."

Christianity's principles of "loving one's neighbor" and placing the care of others before one's own interests were, in many ways, paradoxical, because many wars were fought in later periods in the name of Christianity. Ironically, this created large numbers of casualties and increased the need for expert nursing care. The influence of Christian teachings on the healing work of nurses was extremely pervasive. During the last centuries of the Roman Empire nursing came to be seen as a self-effacing, admirable, and often heroic pursuit.

The Deaconesses of Rome

During the first four centuries A.D., groups of aristocratic women came to embrace the teachings of the church, and the ideals of charitable work. They called themselves "deaconesses," which translates as "ministers." In the early church their role was to assist in baptisms and to visit the poor and sick. They became expert carers and developed nursing practice into a serious discipline for the first time.

Many early leaders of the movement, such as Phebe and Irene, came to be recognized as saints by the Catholic Church. But perhaps the most famous of its members was St Fabiola, whose poignant story has survived in Christian legend.

St Fabiola (d.A.D. 399)

A noblewoman from a patrician Roman family, St Fabiola is said to have endured a miserable arranged marriage at an early age to an abusive husband. Most women in her position at that time would not have taken action, but Fabiola, a well-educated woman of great strength of character, took the unusual and brave step of divorcing her husband and forming a relationship with another man. Her membership of the Christian Church meant that she was unable to marry again while her first husband was still living, and her relationship with her second partner was never formally recognized.

Despite this, Fabiola's religion remained very important to her. After the death of her partner, she made a great impression on her fellow Romans by dressing in rags and undergoing the humiliating process of "public penance." She then used her wealth to help the sick and the poor, founding the first Christian hospital in the world. Fabiola nursed the sickest individuals herself, making a point of dressing the most hideous infected sores and wounds. This brought her celebrity status. By the fourth century A.D. many deaconess movements in the Western Roman Empire had taken the name "matrons." Fabiola joined one such group, which brought her to the attention of the influential St Jerome. She spent time nursing in the Christian hospice in Bethlehem and founded a hospice for pilgrims in Italy.

Opposite:
One of the most famous deaconesses, Fabiola is regarded as the founder of the first Christian hospital in Europe.

The Dark Ages and Medieval Times

The fall of the Roman Empire was followed by several centuries in which people struggled to begin to reconstruct the civilizations they had lost. These centuries are known collectively as the Dark Ages, because very few written records were kept. Most of what we know about these times was recorded by members of religious orders who managed to keep knowledge and learning alive. They also established hospitals where the skills of caring for the frail and elderly were preserved, though in these dark times more emphasis was placed on securing salvation than on health. By the Middle Ages, civilization had begun to recover, and medieval Europe saw the emergence of two movements: women healers within rural societies, and nurses who belonged to religious orders.

WOMEN HEALERS

In the Middle Ages, under the influence of the Catholic Church, the emphasis on curing disease by banishing evil spirits from the body was seen as a threat to the Church's monopoly of spiritual power. Shaman-type healers, therefore, became a thing of the past and rural societies saw an increase in the number of women healers, who offered advice on treatments—particularly herbal medications—as well as nursing care. For many women this healing role simply evolved from what were seen as their normal duties of caring for children, and sick and frail members of their family.

Women healers had no formal education and for this reason were viewed with some suspicion. But although they were, in many ways, the natural successors of shamans, for the most part they avoided the spiritual emphases of their forbears and used a more practical application of their knowledge. Their work might involve ritual and magic, but these elements were carried out in secret. Women healers preserved and handed down knowledge of herbs and other medicinal plants and crystals. Most villages had one "wise woman" who held this knowledge. As she grew older, she selected an apprentice—a younger woman—who she trained in the arts of healing. In this way, knowledge and skill were handed down from expert to novice for generations.

Because healers taught many of their arts in secret, they evaded the two main forms of power that existed in medieval Europe—the patriarchal power of the family and the spiritual power of the Church. The healer was under the power of neither, yet she was valued for the efficacy of her remedies.

Right:
St Sebastian Tended by St Irene and the Holy Women (c.1625) by Georges de la Tour. In the Middle Ages, nursing the sick was seen as a self-denying and redemptive practice. Facing the horrors and rigors of nursing those maimed by battle and disease could offer the living a path to salvation.

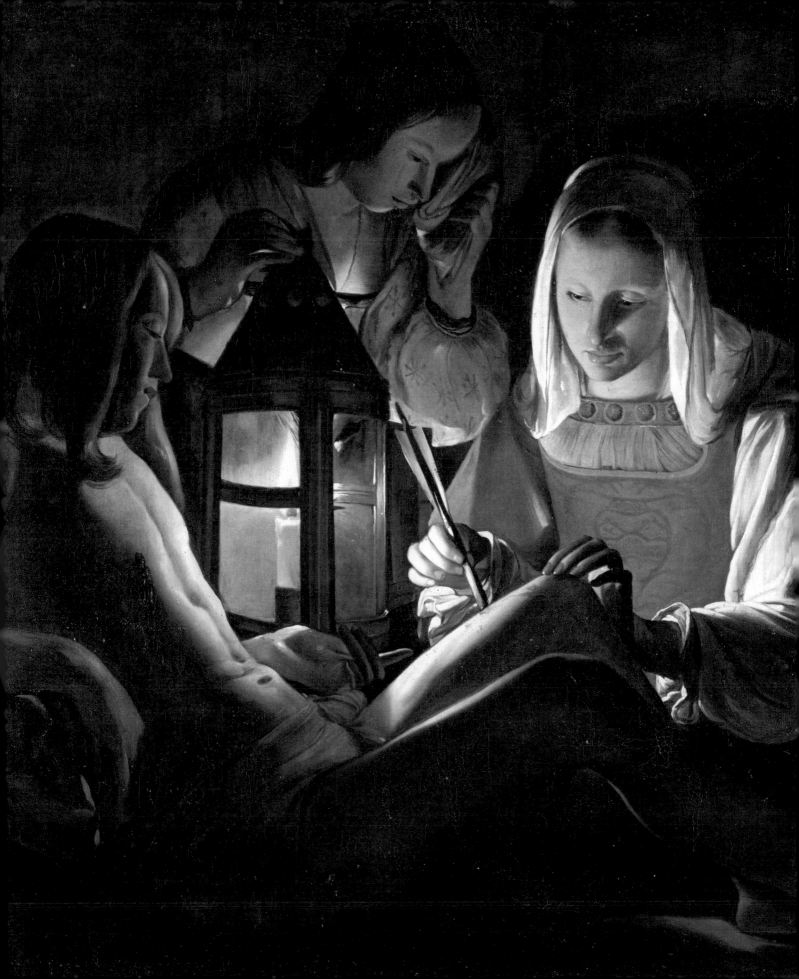

RELIGIOUS AND SECULAR ORDERS

The Middle Ages saw the flourishing of a great monastic movement throughout Europe, and religious orders became an important feature of medieval society. These regular orders were closed. Their members lived a "cloistered" life away from the world and took strict vows of poverty, chastity, and obedience. Within these traditional orders, many of which went on to establish hospitals, nursing was learned as part of the process by which an individual moved from postulant, through novitiate to sister.

Another type of religious movement associated with nursing emerged in the later Middle Ages: the rise of secular orders in which members, although notionally part of a community, lived in the world rather than removed from it. They moved through the streets of medieval and early modern cities,

going into the houses of the sick poor and offering care and comfort. These orders were frequently referred to as "tertiaries." Tertiary orders were founded for laypeople who did not want to be members of enclosed religious orders but did want to devote their lives to good works. They lived apparently ordinary lives "in the world," but their time was spent in works of charity and many of them became expert healers. The most famous tertiaries were St Francis and St Dominic. Their orders attracted the attention of many wealthy and aristocratic men and women who felt moved by a religious faith to renounce their wealth and care for the sick.

Nursing came to be closely associated with saintliness, largely because nurses themselves were seen as heroic. Like the martyrs who died for their beliefs, they put themselves in danger and risked their lives. Unlike the martyrs, however, they did work that was often instrumental in saving the lives of others, working closely with the injured on the battlefield and with the victims of epidemics.

Hildegard of Bingen (1098–1179)

The Abbess Hildegard of Bingen was a remarkable woman who combined the dedication and nursing skills of a nun with the knowledge and acumen of a woman healer. Hildegard was extremely clever. She wrote treatises on healing and natural science and her understanding of nature meant that she had a wealth of knowledge of the herbal and chemical remedies of her day. Recognized as a "mystic," Hildegard is said to have had visions from God, which she wrote down or dictated.

Her unusual powers appear to have arisen from a difficult early life. She was a "sickly" child who was not expected to survive childhood, and it has been suggested that she suffered from severe migraine attacks, which were the origin of her visions. Hildegard became the Prioress of Disibodenberg, a Benedictine convent in the Palatine Forest (now part of Germany), in 1136, but moved her nuns to the independent Rupertsberg Convent at Bingen in 1150.

Right:
Page from a medieval illuminated manuscript, showing Hildegard of Bingen (bottom right-hand corner). Hildegard's approach to healing as a natural and holistic process has led to her being seen as an early exponent of nursing knowledge and practice.

St Elizabeth of Hungary (1207–1231)

Born in Hungary, Elizabeth was a princess who married Ludwig of Thuringia (which is now part of Germany), at the age of fourteen. Despite her position at court, she built a number of hospitals and often worked in them herself, nursing the sick with her own hands. When her husband died in the Crusades, Elizabeth was forced out of her castle and became a member of the Franciscan tertiary order, founding the Franciscan hospital at Marburg. Elizabeth never enjoyed good health herself, yet she worked hard caring for others. She died at the age of twenty-four.

St Catherine of Siena (1347–1380)

Catherine Benincasa was born in 1347, in Siena, Italy, the daughter of a cloth-dyer, and the last of twenty-five siblings. At the age of six, she had a vision that made her determined to devote her life to the service of God. When she reached her teens, her family tried to persuade her to marry, but she refused. She joined the Dominican order and dedicated her life to nursing the sick poor, choosing to care personally for those with the most severe and horrible diseases. She and her followers nursed many plague victims, and she is said to have stayed with patients throughout their illness and then buried them, digging their graves with her own hands. Others she managed to save by her good nursing care. She gained a reputation for supernatural cures, and came to be held in awe because of her own survival through the nursing of so many dangerously ill patients.

Because Catherine seemed to be so unusual there were those who were afraid of her. She was accused of heresy, but cleared of the charge in 1374. She began to gain a reputation for settling disputes and campaigned actively to heal the political schism that had emerged in the Catholic Church, becoming highly influential among popes and many ruling Italian families. Said to have been unable to write, she may have dictated her many literary works to a secretary. Catherine died of a stroke at the age of thirty-three.

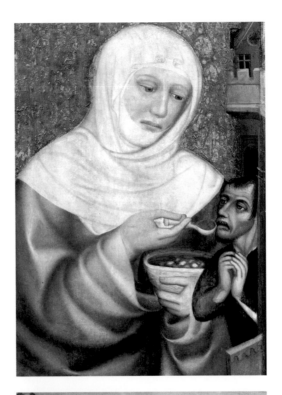

Left:
St Elizabeth of Hungary *(fourteenth century) by Theodoricus of Prague. St Elizabeth is shown feeding a pauper.*

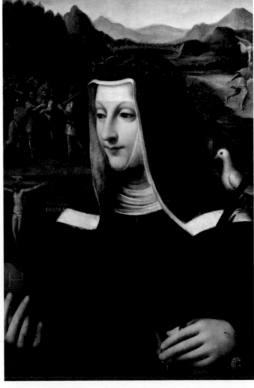

Left:
Fifteenth-century votive painting of St Catherine of Siena. The dove on her shoulder symbolizes Catherine's role as peacemaker.

MILITARY NURSING ORDERS

Nowhere was the heroic image of nursing expressed more clearly or determinedly than among the military nursing orders that emerged during the Wars of the Crusades in the eleventh, twelfth, and thirteenth centuries. These orders, known as "brotherhoods," were of great significance because they offered men a healing role, and asserted that nursing could be a masculine pursuit. The brotherhoods also accepted women, but, as was typical in a patriarchal society, the female and male sections were segregated. Women who nursed were seen as subordinate to the men, who both fought *and* nursed.

Military nursing orders upheld the medieval ideals of chivalry, heroism, and charity, and became celebrated for their courage and compassion. They also became wealthy from the donations of grateful noblemen and royal families, amassing lands and treasure, and building huge hospitals in the Holy Land and on main routes between Europe and the Middle East.

The most significant of the military orders was probably the Order of the Knights Hospitallers of St John of Jerusalem, with its female branch, the Hospitaller Dames. The origins of the order are obscure but it is clear that in the eleventh century members decided to take strict religious vows, and began to wear long black robes with white Maltese crosses embroidered onto them. The order was formally named and established in 1113, and, at the end of the Crusades, set up its main base on the island of Rhodes, but was forced out by invading Turks. In 1530 it was given a base on Malta, where it established its most magnificent hospital at Valetta in 1575. Today, the Order of St John of Jerusalem has its base in London and provides important first-aid training through centers in Europe and America.

Right:

Lithograph showing the gate of the hospital of the Knights of St John of Jerusalem. The Knights Hospitallers were formed to offer care and support to those who were injured or made ill as a result of their activities in the Crusades. Their most important hospitals were therefore situated in the Holy Land itself (as shown here, in Jerusalem), or en route to Europe.

Opposite:

Hospital run by the Order of St John of Jerusalem. Knights Hospitallers are shown nursing the patients.

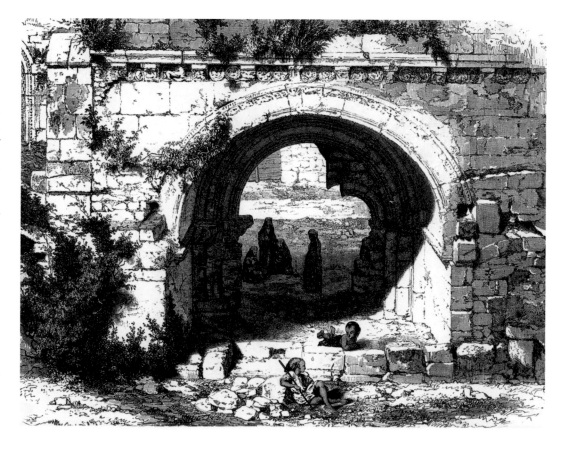

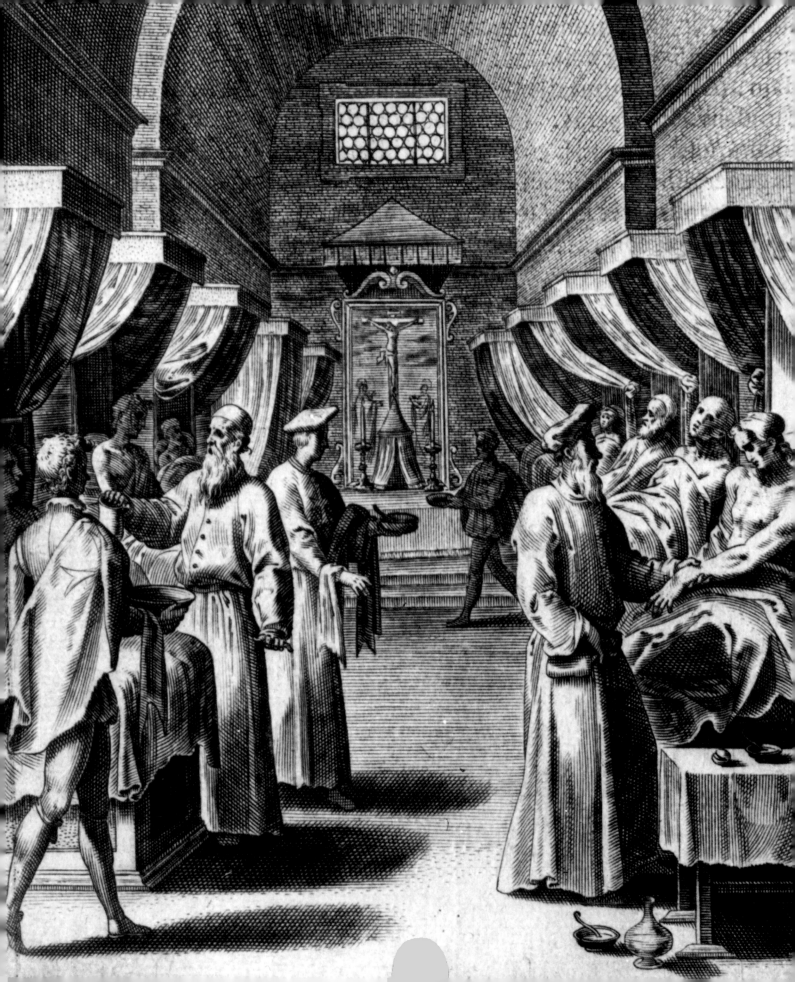

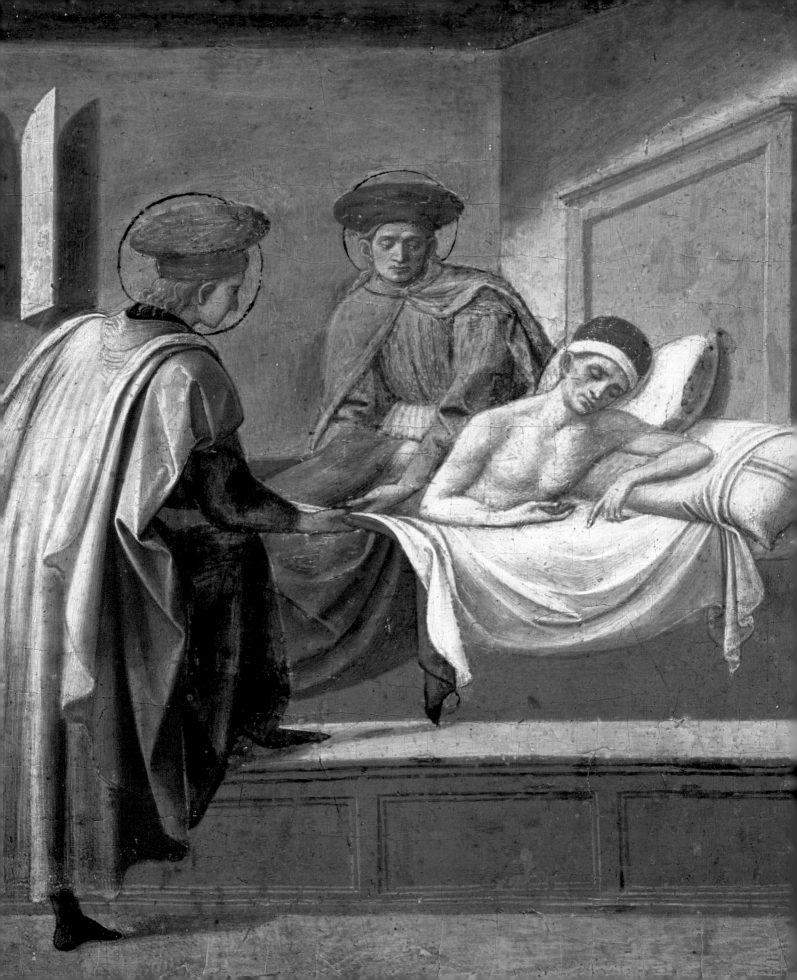

The Early Modern Period (c.1450–1800)

As the Middle Ages gave way to the Early Modern period, nursing knowledge continued to be learned as part of an oral tradition; nursing practice was learned by direct hands-on experience. Women healers passed on their wisdom and expertise by taking on young apprentices who they instructed in their art. As civilized arts such as reading and writing became more widespread—first in religious houses and later in society at large— individuals made a point of recording important herbal remedies and techniques for caring for the sick. However, the art of nursing was something that could only be passed on from teacher to pupil through direct experience. Only by working with an expert nurse could one learn the secrets of care, comfort, and healing.

INDEPENDENT HEALERS

Nurses who practiced in rural areas became highly regarded and respected for the skills and knowledge they accumulated. These were of real practical value at a time when medicine was seen as a highly esoteric pursuit, studied at a few extremely elite universities, and practiced by individuals who often took pains to protect themselves by keeping a distance from their patients. During the great European plagues of the sixteenth and seventeenth centuries, some physicians attended patients— when they visited them at all—wearing huge masks, their faces hidden behind the various protective herbs and chemicals that were packed into great beak-shaped contraptions. It was local "handywomen" and members of religious orders who practised hands-on healing for the acutely ill and dying. Yet many women healers found themselves in danger during the craze that led to massive witch-hunts in the sixteenth and seventeenth centuries, when both Catholic and Protestant churches became determined to pursue those they saw as deriving their power from pacts with the devil. Ironically, it was often the women who seemed, by their knowledge and wisdom of healing, to hold this type of power who became the victims of what was really an epidemic of religious paranoia.

Many women in rural areas—both ladies-of-the-manor and poor "wise women"—did become knowledgeable in herbal medicine, but there was no guarantee that their knowledge would be preserved. The nursing care within a household was generally in the hands of the female "head," though the nursing itself was often delegated to servants. Under these circumstances, the development of the art of nursing could only be passed on by unreliable, ad hoc processes such as word-of-mouth.

Opposite:
SS. Cosmas and Damian Healing the Sick *(fifteenth century) by Francesco Pesellino. Twin brothers and famous members of a tertiary order, St Cosmas and St Damian are shown practicing the art of hands-on healing.*

THE NEW NURSING ORDERS

In the sixteenth century, a powerful religious movement, the Protestant Reformation, divided Europe. Some nation-states adopted the Protestant religions advocated by reformers such as Martin Luther, John Calvin, and others who were highly critical of the Catholic Church. In these states Catholic institutions were outlawed and new state-run churches were established.

In England, the formation of the Anglican Church was accompanied by the dissolution of the monasteries. All monastic institutions, and most of the hospitals they supported, were abolished. Even though some important institutions, such as St Bartholomew's Hospital in London, were preserved under new, secular leadership, the dissolution of the monasteries was a devastating blow for the organized care of the sick in England—a blow from which it was not to recover fully until the nineteenth century.

States whose rulers decided they would remain Catholic also underwent important change in a series of movements that came collectively to be known as the Counter-Reformation. There was a turning-back to what were seen as the original values of the Catholic Church. This meant that "good works" such as healing were once again valued. New nursing orders emerged in Catholic countries under the guiding influence of the Counter-Reformation.

Nursing was seen as a caring art. The aim of the nurse was to make the patient "whole"—to heal him physically, emotionally, and spiritually. In Europe, this caring ethos developed rapidly within Catholic religious communities. Until the reforms of the nineteenth century, the only really effective nursing care was offered by religious orders. Their members usually had some education, received an apprenticeship training from experienced mentors, and were serious in their desire to help their patients.

Camillus of Lellis (1550–1614)

One classic story of a Renaissance male nurse is that of Camillus, born in Bucchianico in southern Italy. His mother died when he was very young and his father was a soldier who was rarely home. Camillus endured a lonely and neglected childhood and a troubled youth. He joined the Venetian army at a very early age, and became addicted to gambling. It is not known what drew him to hospital work, except that he had severe abscesses on his feet caused by injuries received in the army, and so his first encounter with nursing must have been as a patient. His first experience of work for the Hospital for Incurables in Rome was disastrous, and he was dismissed for gambling, but he later rejoined the staff of the hospital, this time remaining to become its director.

Camillus decided to found his own brotherhood, the Ministers of the Sick, which became known as the Camillians. Its purpose was to nurse those suffering from hopeless injuries or epidemic diseases. The Camillians became famous for their willingness to work with plague victims who everyone else shunned in fear. A special group within the order worked with these hopeless cases, and became known as the "Brothers of the Good Death." Interestingly, Camillus himself became known as a miracle-healer for personally bringing some of these victims back from the brink of death. It was probably, in fact, good nursing care, rather than miracles that saved these patients. Camillus himself endured severe disability throughout his life as a result of his war injuries. He was canonized in 1746.

Right:
Eighteenth-century marble statue of Camillus of Lellis, by Petrus Pacilli, in St Peter's Basilica, Rome.

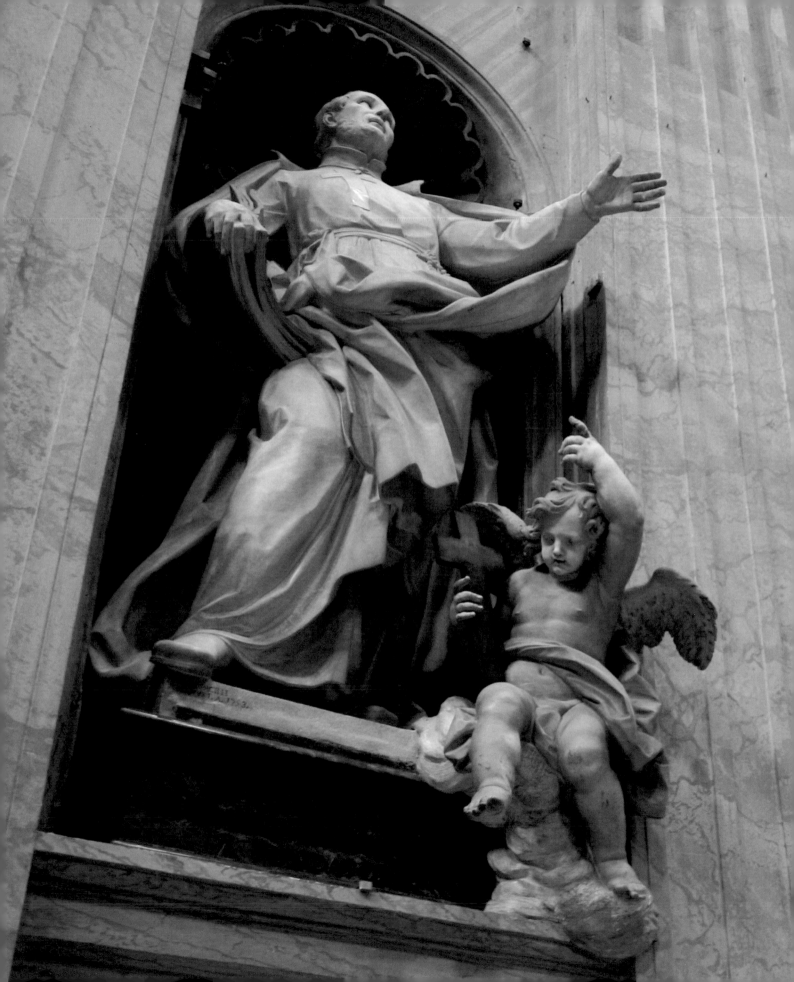

The Daughters of Charity

Many of the new religious orders that came into existence throughout Europe dedicated themselves to care of the sick. Among the most important was the Daughters of Charity, a movement that emerged in France in the early seventeenth century. It was founded in 1634 by a Catholic priest, Vincent de Paul, working closely with a noblewoman, Louise de Marillac. The son of a wealthy peasant, de Paul was born in central France, educated at the University of Toulouse, and ordained a priest in 1600. In 1605, when on a voyage from Marseille, he was captured by Turkish pirates and sold into slavery. He gained his release by converting his owner to Christianity.

Louise de Marillac (1591–1660)

De Paul met Louise de Marillac in 1625 and together they decided to found a sisterhood for the care of the sick. Louise had been born to the mistress of a prominent nobleman. Her mother died soon after giving birth, and her father's family cared for and educated her, but never accepted or acknowledged her as a family member. She accepted an arranged marriage in 1613, even though she really wanted to enter a convent. Twelve years later, she was widowed, and decided to use her new-found freedom to care for the poor. In 1633, using funds provided by a group known as the Ladies of Charity, de Paul and Marillac worked to develop a community of nurses they named the Daughters of Charity. Louise brought a group of poor countrywomen together into her own home and taught them how to provide care for the sick. The education provided for these women became more sophisticated, and the movement spread rapidly. By the time Louise died, in 1660, there were more than forty houses in France, and Daughters of Charity were caring for the sick poor in their own homes throughout the poorest neighborhoods of Paris. Eventually, the Daughters of Charity were asked to provide the nursing care at the oldest and largest Paris hospital, the Hôtel Dieu. They extended their work across France and developed nursing in hospitals, prisons, orphanages, and other institutions. The Daughters of Charity dressed in blue-gray habits, and became known as the Grey

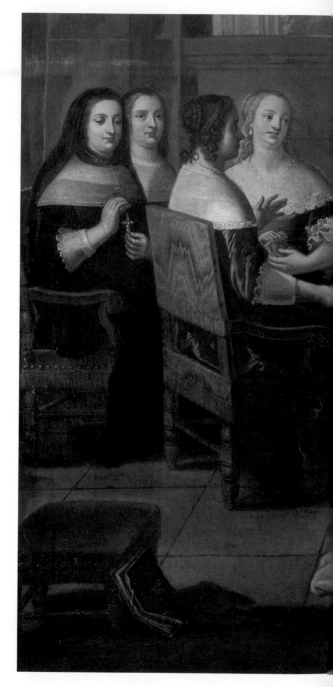

Nuns, even though theirs was not a closed religious order. Their vows were simple, and they enjoyed greater freedom than any regular order of nuns. Their large white "cornette" headdresses made them instantly recognizable.

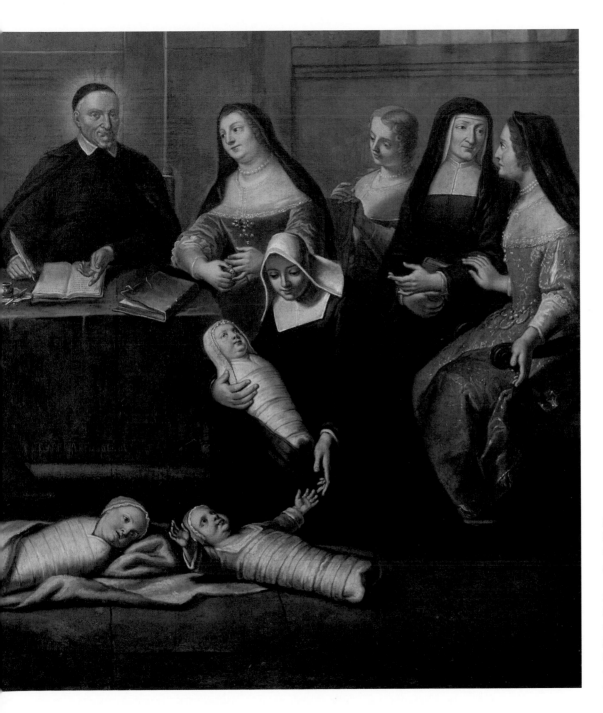

Left:
St Vincent de Paul and
the Sisters of Charity
*(c.1729), by Jean Andre.
Vincent de Paul is shown
in the center, surrounded
by members of the Ladies
of Charity—a rich,
philanthropic organization
that supported the
development of the
Daughters of Charity.*

NURSING IN THE NEW WORLD

The Early Modern period has been seen as an age of exploration. Great seafaring nations such as England, France, Spain, and Portugal sent expeditions to all parts of the globe. Explorers like Christopher Columbus and Jean Cabot navigated the Atlantic Ocean, hoping to find a shortcut to the East Indies. Instead they discovered the completely "New World" of North America. The Spanish and Portuguese, on similar expeditions, conquered and colonized South and Central America. Nurses rapidly became part of these early colonizing societies, through Catholic religious orders. Often, their primary mission was to Christianize "native" populations, and as part of this they established great hospitals and schools.

Jeanne Mance (1606–1673)

The Grey Nuns were one of the first nursing groups to move across the Atlantic to the New World. One of the most romantic figures of Canadian nursing, Jeanne Mance, learned to nurse at l'Hôpital de la Charité at Langres, France, an establishment formed in 1638 and modeled on the work of the Daughters of Charity. In 1640, Jeanne was invited by the wealthy Madame Angélique de Bullion to establish a hospital in "New France"—later to be known as Quebec. She departed from La Rochelle in 1641 as part of a group led by the French military officer Sieur de Maisonneuve, which planted a European colony known as Ville Marie on the island of Montreal. The first hospital was a small hut inside the fort, where Jeanne nursed the wounded from skirmishes between the French colonizers and the local Iroquois tribe, who did not appreciate the establishment of a European settlement in their territory.

In 1645 a new hospital was built and it appeared that the colony might become more settled. However, in 1651, fighting intensified and Jeanne and her assistants were kept busy caring for wounded men, including patients who had been scalped and who were nursed back to health by Jeanne's nurses. On one occasion the fort's garrison was saved by a warning from Jeanne that a band of Iroquois was approaching. For two years after this,

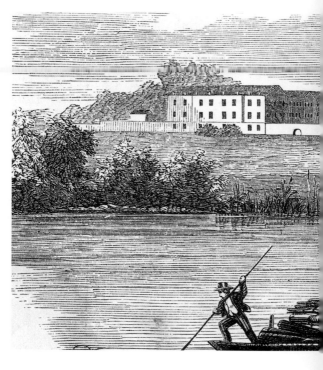

her hospital became an outpost occupied by soldiers, while she and her staff were confined inside the fort itself.

In 1657, Jeanne was joined by three members of the St Joseph Hospitallers of La Flèche, from France, one of whom, Judith Moreau de Bresoles, took over the running of the newly built Hôtel Dieu.

Nursing in French Canada

The Hôtel Dieu of Montreal was not the first hospital to be established in French Canada. The Hôtel Dieu of Quebec, founded by the white-robed Augustinian Nursing Sisters from Dieppe in Normandy, France, was established in 1639. These nuns were members of a cloistered order, bound by strict vows, and they personified the self-sacrifice of the regular clergy. They arrived after a difficult voyage, in the middle of an epidemic, and were immediately faced with having to look after hundreds of infectious patients, many of whom had to be cared for in hastily built huts outside the hospital walls. The Hôtel Dieu in Quebec thrived. In 1788 Marie-Angelique Viger (Saint-Martin)

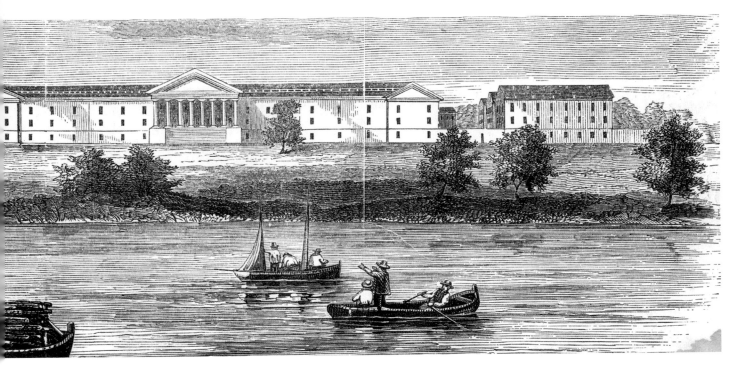

became the apothecary, and was said to have saved many lives, including that of a patient on whom she performed a leg amputation.

The women who established nursing care within the large hospitals of French Canada were intrepid pioneers. They were also diplomats, unconscious of their power to heal not only the bodies of individual colonists, but also the rifts between those who fought for mastery and control. In the 1760s, when the English conquered Quebec and made it part of a united Canada, it was the French nursing sisters who acted as a vital link between the two opposing sides. They cared for French, British, Iroquois, and Algonquin alike, and, by their humanitarian efforts, offered a means for rapprochement. Their vital work with the victims of the frequent epidemics that struck French Canada was an important force in healing and uniting the region. The Augustinian Nuns of Quebec City and the Grey Nuns of Montreal did important work that went largely unacknowledged. This is, perhaps, typical of nurses throughout history, who have worked behind the scenes, looking for neither fame nor recognition.

Nursing in North America

The Pilgrim Fathers, who founded some of the earliest European settlements in what is now the USA, took with them individuals known to be skilled in caring for the sick. The earliest group of settlers is believed to have taken a Dutch deaconess-nurse with them when they departed from Holland. One of the earliest hospitals in America was founded in 1658 by the West India Company in New Amsterdam, later to be renamed New York City. This hospital was linked to the poorhouse and was to be the predecessor of the famous Bellevue Hospital. The "Charity" of New Orleans, run by Sisters of Charity, was founded in 1720 and became the city hospital in 1811.

In the eighteenth and early nineteenth centuries, many American hospitals, like their European counterparts, were connected with poorhouses. They were badly funded, and nursing care was offered by untrained paupers who were themselves destitute. The scene was set in both Protestant Europe and the North American continent for another much needed regeneration of nursing.

Above:

The Philadelphia General Hospital, originally known as the Blockley, was founded as an almshouse in 1730, when it was run by its pauper inmates. It became a hospital in 1816. In 1832, nursing here was briefly put into the hands of a group of Sisters of Charity from Emmitsburg, who nursed the victims of a severe cholera epidemic and temporarily brought order to the demoralized institution.

Uniforms

Nurses' uniforms evolved over time. Early healers did not wear any specific form of clothing designed to set them apart. In the Middle Ages, when religious orders began to involve themselves in caring for the sick, the nun's habit began to be clearly associated with nursing work. Nursing evolved as a profession and a discipline in the nineteenth century. Yet the flowing robes of the nun continued to wield a strong influence over the development of nurses' uniforms for many years.

As cadres of nurses developed in hospitals throughout the world, they designed uniforms that would identify them with their own particular institution. Pride in belonging to highly respected hospitals led to the development of sometimes flamboyant uniforms with puffed sleeves and full skirts. These were nevertheless still essentially practical in design, and bore at least a passing resemblance to the domestic servant's dress.

Color and style were used symbolically: white for hygiene and cleanliness; blue for purity; pink for femininity. One of the most striking uniforms of the late nineteenth and early twentieth centuries was the Red Cross nurse's uniform, upon which was emblazoned the powerful symbol of the red cross, denoting humanitarian aid to the battle wounded on all sides of any conflict.

Uniforms were a combination of the practical, the political, and the symbolic—bands, stripes, and colors were used to differentiate between ranks. In the late twentieth century there was a deliberate move toward breaking down barriers, as nurses began to wear scrubs. The value of such clothing was seen to lie in its practicality and unisex nature. Scrubs were not popular with everyone, though. Many believed that they were too similar to pajamas or children's clothes. Today's uniforms are more carefully designed and are regaining their symbolic status. Yet, some of the more modern nursing roles are not associated with uniform at all. Many nurse-specialists and nurse-consultants wear ordinary smart clothes, sometimes protected by a white coat—perhaps indicating that nursing has come "full circle" back to its roots as a broader-based and more independent healing discipline.

From left to right:
Nineteenth-century uniforms of nurses from France, England, USA, and Australia.

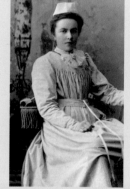 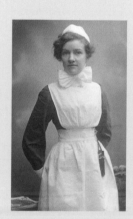 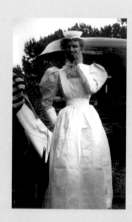 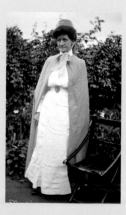

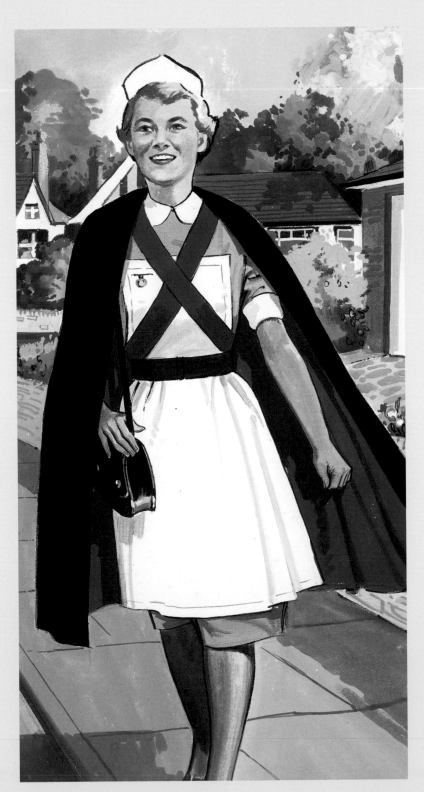

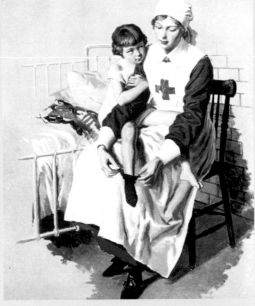

Left:
Illustration of a mid-twentieth century British nurse in uniform, taken from the English children's educational series of Look and Learn *books.*

Above:
A Red Cross nurse and child as depicted by the 1920s Italian artist Fortunino Matania.

Below:
A 21st-century nurse in scrubs.

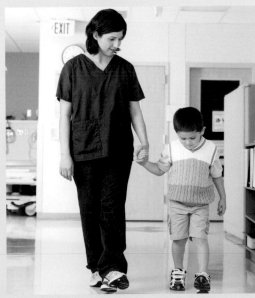

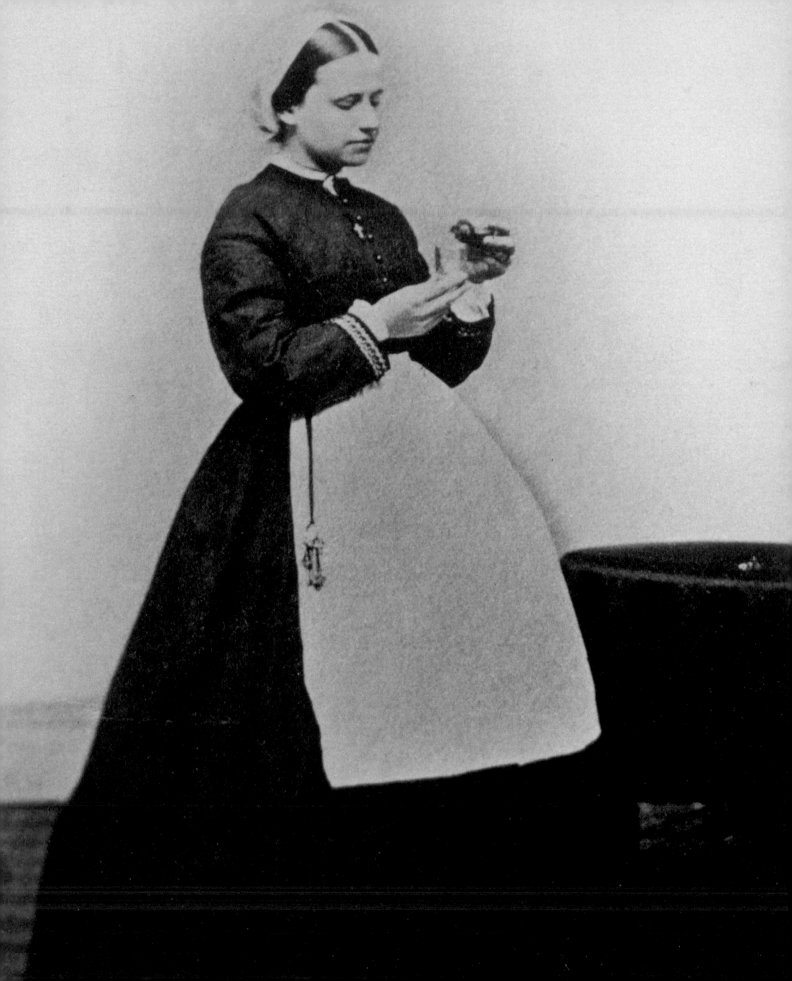

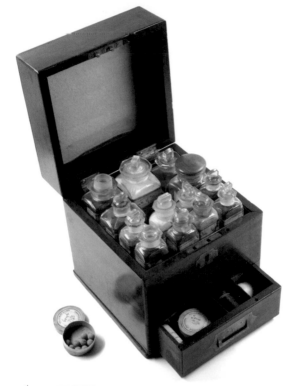

THE NINETEENTH CENTURY

During the nineteenth century, nursing changed
from an expression of religious piety to a professional
discipline. This extraordinary transition was shaped
by memorable events and individuals, as nurses took
an increasing role in public health care and the fight
against disease.

2

From Nun to Professional Nurse

In Catholic countries nursing continued to develop, but in countries
that had adopted the Protestant religion during the sixteenth-century
Reformation, the Early Modern period had been a dark time for nurses. In
rural areas women healers were often the backbone of health care, yet they
were viewed as outcasts and sometimes persecuted as witches. At the same
time, there were no monastic or tertiary orders in which the knowledge
and skill of nursing could be kept alive. In England, Wales, and Scotland, in
parts of continental Europe such as Germany and the Netherlands, and
in Scandinavian countries such as Norway and Sweden, there was no real
skilled nursing care. Many women in rural areas did become knowledgeable
in herbal medicine, but there was no guarantee that their knowledge would
be preserved.

THE NEED FOR REFORM

By the early nineteenth century it was beginning
to be realized in Protestant countries that care of
the sick was a neglected field. During the "shock
era" of the 1830s and 1840s, industrialization,
which had made a slow and tentative start in the
late eighteenth century, advanced rapidly—too
rapidly for local communities to cope with its
consequences. The growth of factories for the mass
production of goods meant that there was a migration of workers from country districts to towns and
cities. Urban centers grew rapidly, outstripping
their supplies of food and water and outgrowing
the availability of adequate housing. Many people
in these cities lived in a state of abject poverty in
cramped, inadequately ventilated tenement apart-
ments, with several individuals sleeping in each
room, breathing the polluted air and drinking the
polluted water created by industrial processes.
Many died during vast epidemics of cholera. People
had lost contact with friends and family who might
have been able to offer them support. They had also
lost contact with those skilled healers who had
been such a feature of rural life.

As so often happens in such circumstances, elite
members of society were slow to recognize the
enormity of the problem, while those who suffered
were helpless to act. Initially a few lone voices from
the middle ranks of society spoke about the need
for reform. Eventually, their cause would be taken
up by wealthy philanthropists, and by some politi-
cians. The first impetus for reform was driven
forward by individuals such as Elizabeth Fry (see
page 38), whose actions were heavily influenced
by Christian piety and a desire to help the poor.
Some of the earliest organized centers of nursing
in Protestant Europe were those created by
"deaconesses" in Germany and Scandinavia.

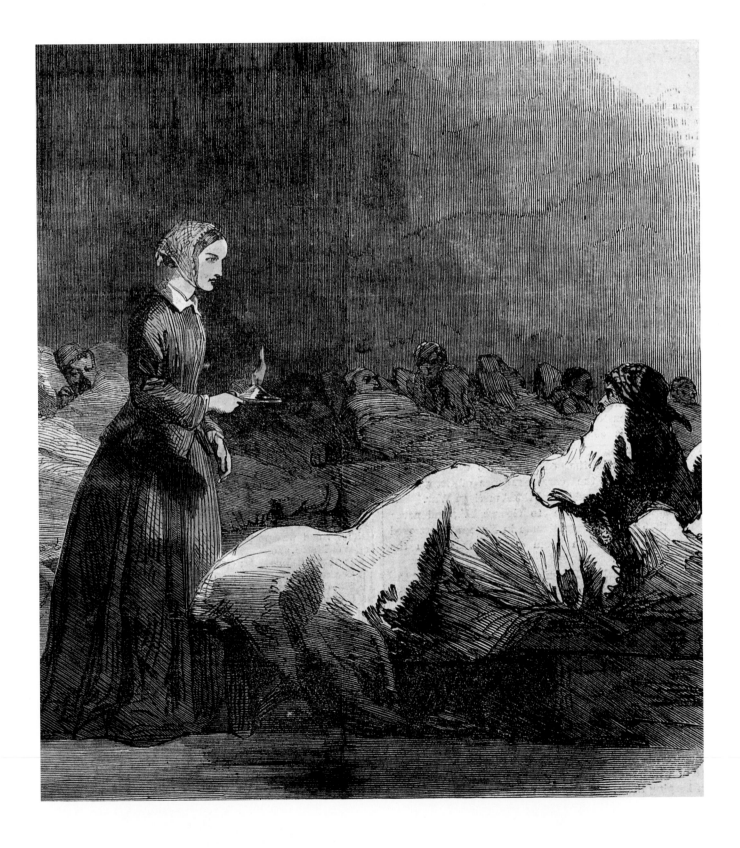

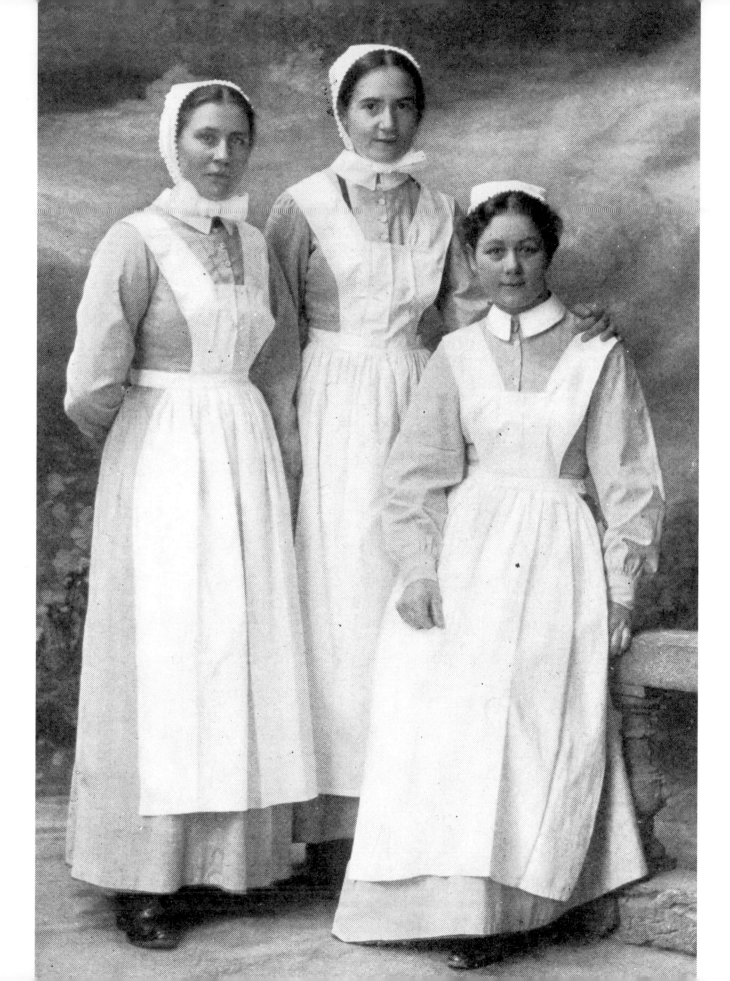

German Deaconesses

Deliberately taking the title adopted by those early Roman noblewomen whose names had gone down in legend, the German deaconesses established themselves in a number of towns and cities, and were among the earliest Protestant sisterhoods.

These groups of women lived a communal life, but did not take vows. Although motivated by religious zeal, they were not bound by any "rule" or "order." They can be seen as part of a movement that deliberately reached back into the past and found a way of creating a bridge to a future in which nursing would be performed, not by nuns controlled by a religious authority, but by independent groups of women professing a worthy art. The religious symbolism adopted by these movements was partly a consequence of a genuine religious faith that drove their actions. However, it was also a more calculated means by which women—who were normally expected to remain in the domestic sphere, and for whom work outside the home was seen as highly suspect—persuaded society that their nursing work was "safe" and "respectable." In this way, they managed to stay within the bounds of acceptability and apparent safety, while actually performing some remarkable and dangerous work.

The most famous of the German deaconess houses was that run by Theodor Fliedner and his wife Friederike at Kaiserswerth in the Rhineland, which had a school, an orphanage, and a hospital. Young women were trained to visit the sick poor in their own homes and offer them nursing care and health advice. Florence Nightingale visited Kaiserswerth when she was grappling with the problems of how to become a nurse in the days before anyone in Britain really knew what that was. She was to be one of many nurse-reformers who visited the Kaiserswerth Institution to learn how to re-create nursing for the nineteenth century.

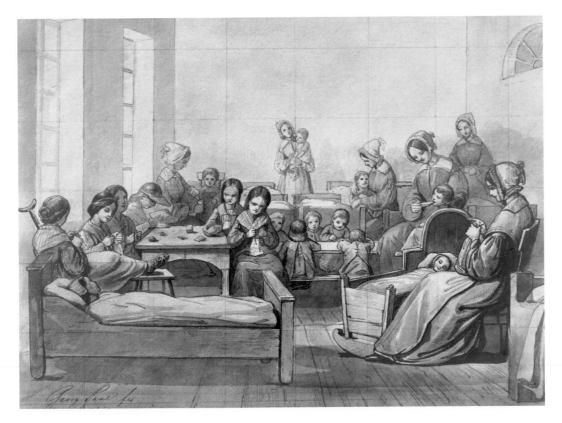

Left:

Kaiserswerth was the most famous and one of the earliest German deaconess houses. As well as a training center for nurses, it was also an orphanage.

Opposite:

Sisters from a deaconess hospital in Stockholm, Sweden.

Elizabeth Fry (1780–1845)

As with so many nursing reformers, it was religious faith that inspired Elizabeth Fry to help the poor. However, in her case, it was not mystical Catholicism but a radical form of Protestantism that drove her work. Elizabeth was a Quaker who believed that God's power could be felt through the words and actions of individual human beings. She came from a wealthy banking family, and enjoyed a comfortable childhood in Norwich, England, but her mother died when she was twelve years old, leaving her as the main carer for her younger brothers and sisters. From the age of eighteen, Elizabeth took a deep interest in the health and welfare of her poorer neighbors, taking them food and clothing and visiting them when they were sick. Such informal visiting was very typical of the ladies of her time. Many of the works of early nineteenth-century novelists such as Jane Austen and George Eliot describe young wealthy gentlewomen visiting the homes of their neighbors and taking an interest in the welfare of the poor. However, Elizabeth soon came to realize that visiting one's neighbors in this way was never really going to change their lives. Indeed, such apparent generosity really just masked the injustice of a society in which some people lived in wealth while others were in abject poverty.

After her marriage, Elizabeth moved with her husband to London, where she became interested in prison reform after seeing the appalling conditions under which female prisoners lived at Newgate prison. After much campaigning, she persuaded the Home Secretary, Robert Peel, to reform the British justice system in 1823. In 1840, Elizabeth established the Institution of Nursing Sisters, which developed one of the earliest training programs for nurses. Young women of lower social classes were given a uniform and underwent a three-month training at Guy's and various other London hospitals. Elizabeth's work had an important influence on Florence Nightingale, who took some of Fry's nurses with her to the Crimea in 1854.

"I believe firmly that all is guided for the best by an invisible power, therefore I do not fear the evils of life so much. I love to feel good—I do what I can to be kind to everybody. I have many faults which I hope in time to overcome."

Elizabeth Fry

Journal entry for May 16, 1797, from Memoir of the Life of Elizabeth Fry, *edited by Katherine Fry and Rachel Cresswell (1847)*

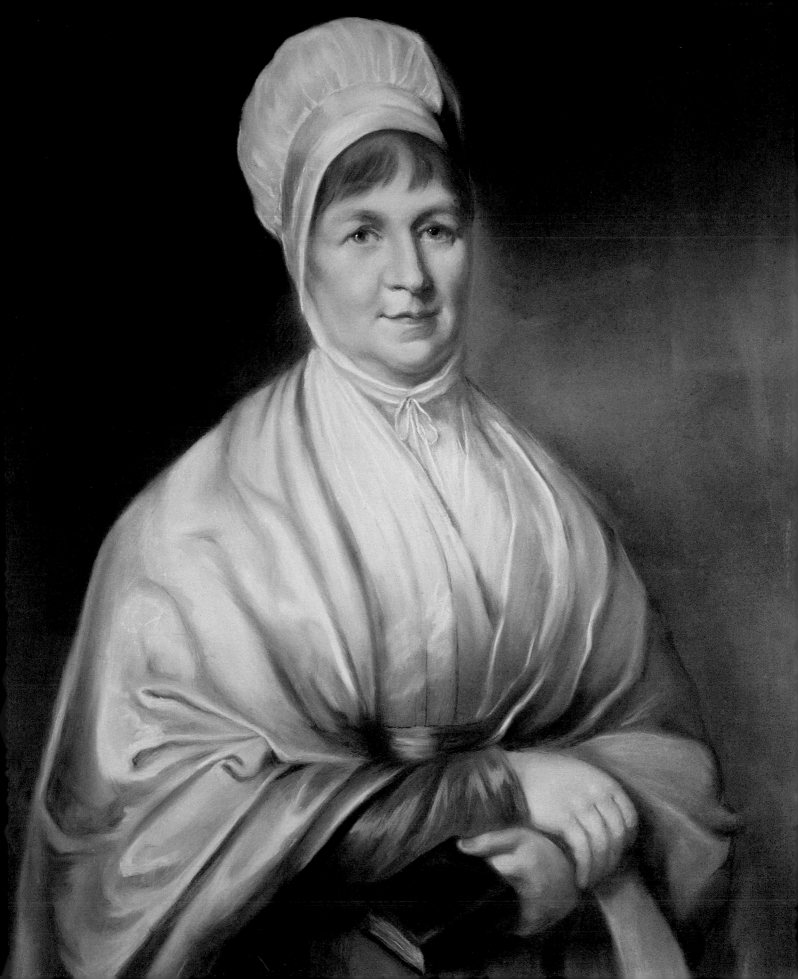

Anglican Sisterhoods in England

The impetus of Elizabeth Fry's work was enough to encourage other women to believe that nursing might be an acceptable social role for educated women. The earliest Anglican nursing sisterhood was the Park Village community, established near Regent's Park, London, England, in 1845. This was followed a few years later by the founding of the Sisters of Mercy (Sellonite Order) in Devonport, England, by Priscilla Lydia Sellon. Both of these sisterhoods, although established within the Protestant Anglican Church, resembled Catholic communities. Some of their members even took vows of poverty, chastity, and obedience. This meant that they were regarded with suspicion by a British society that had only recently offered full citizenship rights to Catholics.

One of the reasons for the early success of St John's House, a sisterhood founded in London in 1848, was its careful avoidance of excessive religious influence of any kind. Another was the patronage of Robert Bentley Todd, a powerful Professor of Anatomy and Physiology at King's College. St John's House was established as both a physical community where its members might choose to live and an educational institution that offered a two-year program of training, including lectures from physicians. It represented an important break with the past. No longer was nursing essentially an expression of religious fervor; it was a profession, based on sound scientific principles and learned within hospital wards.

Mary Jones (1812–1887)

Born in Tamworth, England, in 1812, the daughter of a cabinetmaker, Mary Jones had a considerable influence on the nursing profession. Having joined St John's House in 1848, she was elected its Lady Superintendent in 1853, and trained nurses to accompany Florence Nightingale to the Crimea. In 1856, St John's House took over the nursing duties of King's College Hospital, London, and Mary became Sister-in-Charge of nursing at King's. Ten years later, the scope of St John's increased as the sisters also took charge of nursing at Charing Cross Hospital, London.

Mary established a midwifery-training program at King's College Hospital, which was, unfortunately, closed due to a high mortality rate from infection on the maternity ward. She was one of the first ever Lady Superintendents to insist that the head of nursing in any hospital should have complete control over the nursing work, and resisted all efforts by the St John's Council (all of whom were male) to interfere in any way in the lives and work of the nurses. In fact, it was a dispute with her board that led Mary to resign in 1868 and establish a new community known as the Sisterhood of St Mary and St John located near King's Cross. In 1872, as part of this new venture, she founded the St Joseph's Hospital for Incurables. Mary died of typhoid fever in 1887. She is said to have given great encouragement and support to Florence Nightingale and was one of Florence's most trusted professional allies.

Dorothy Pattison (1832–1878)

Often better known as "Sister Dora," Dorothy Pattison was born in Yorkshire, England. She had no formal education, as her father disapproved of education for women, but with the help of her eldest brother, who attended Oxford University, she developed a learned mind. In 1864, Dorothy joined the Christ Church Anglican Sisterhood at Coatham, and was sent to the Walsall cottage hospital in January 1865. Although virtually self-taught, she rose to become matron of the hospital, and was renowned for her skill and knowledge as a surgical nurse. She learned by attending post-mortems and dissections, and by the end of her career was capable of performing minor surgery. However, when one of the doctors with whom she worked suggested that she ought to train as a doctor, she pointed out that nursing was her preferred form of work.

In 1872, during a fatal colliery disaster, Dorothy stayed at the pit head with the families of victims, offering them her support and care. Because she so obviously cared for the people with whom she worked, she came to be revered as a saint in Walsall.

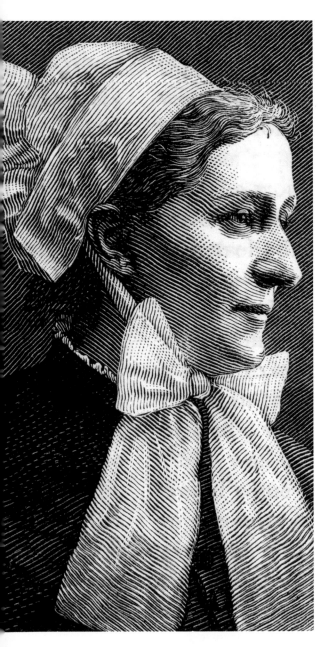

Dorothy was often in conflict with her sisterhood. On one occasion she nursed the victims of a smallpox epidemic against their orders. In 1878 she made a tour of a number of European hospitals and visited London, where she observed the work of Joseph Lister, and ordered the purchase of equipment to make antiseptic surgery possible in Walsall.

SISTERHOODS IN NORTH AMERICA

In the nineteenth century North America was seen as a land of freedom. Europeans wanting to escape poverty, persecution, or both, migrated across the Atlantic to found new communities in the West. Because of its origins as a refuge from bigotry and persecution of any kind, America was a place where Catholic or Protestant nursing sisterhoods could equally easily be established. The French movement of the Daughters of Charity inspired the development of a new movement in Emmitsburg, Maryland, in 1809. It was headed by Elizabeth Ann Seton, and was known as the Sisters of Charity of St Joseph. Forty years later, in 1849, nurses from Kaiserswerth in Germany established a deaconess house in Pittsburgh, Pennsylvania. Sisters of Charity nursed during the cholera epidemics in the cities of New York, Philadelphia, and Baltimore, under the direct control of the city authorities.

In the rapidly growing "new world" of North America, many individuals depended on the sort of informal networks of care that had been important in Europe until the breakdown of community life during the Industrial Revolution. Private nursing was often of good quality. Communities had their own nurses who were recognized as experts in the arts of healing and were trusted figures.

Later in the nineteenth century, Linda Richards (see page 65) was to comment that:

"Those women, who by their kindness of heart and cheerful service were called the born nurses, were by no means untrained. Experience, which is an excellent teacher, together with the instruction of older women and of the family doctor, provided a practical and efficient training. A love of the work and a desire to alleviate suffering made most of them excellent nurses."

Left:
Dorothy Pattison gave her name to the "Sister Dora" cap, which she is seen wearing here.

Military Nursing

At the beginning of the nineteenth century, Europe was a fractured, fragmented collection of nation-states, each anxiously defending its territory from threats outside its borders. Conflicts had been frequent in the Early Modern period, and the religious split caused by the Reformation had added a layer of ideology—and sometimes fanaticism—to the passions that fueled Europe's frequent wars. As the century opened, the Revolutionary and Napoleonic wars, in which an authoritarian state was attempting to expand its boundaries and create an empire at the expense of its neighbors, were in full swing. The people of these states had grown accustomed to conflict and violence, and yet the warfare of the nineteenth century was also new and different, as weaponry became increasingly advanced.

CARE OF THE WOUNDED

The invention of increasingly destructive weaponry meant that battles inevitably caused large numbers of casualties. Because standing armies were large, a set-piece battle was likely to end with many hundreds of wounded and dying men lying on the battlefield. The care of these men was usually woefully inadequate. Any relief they were offered came from two groups: military orderlies, chosen from among their own ranks, and female camp-followers. Although the latter were viewed as uniformly disreputable, many were, in fact, the wives and sweethearts of soldiers, who followed armies and cared for their wounded out of loyalty, compassion, and patriotism. However, there was nothing remotely resembling an organized military nursing service. It is largely for this reason that the work of Florence Nightingale in the Crimea in the mid-century has typically been presented, by those who like to see history as progress, as a transformative and revolutionary force, not just in the history of nursing, but also in the advance of humanitarianism.

"Others have described the horrors of those fatal trenches; but their real history has never been written, and perhaps it is as well that so harrowing a tale should be left in oblivion."

Mary Seacole

Extract from The Wonderful Adventures of Mrs Seacole in Many Lands *(1857)*

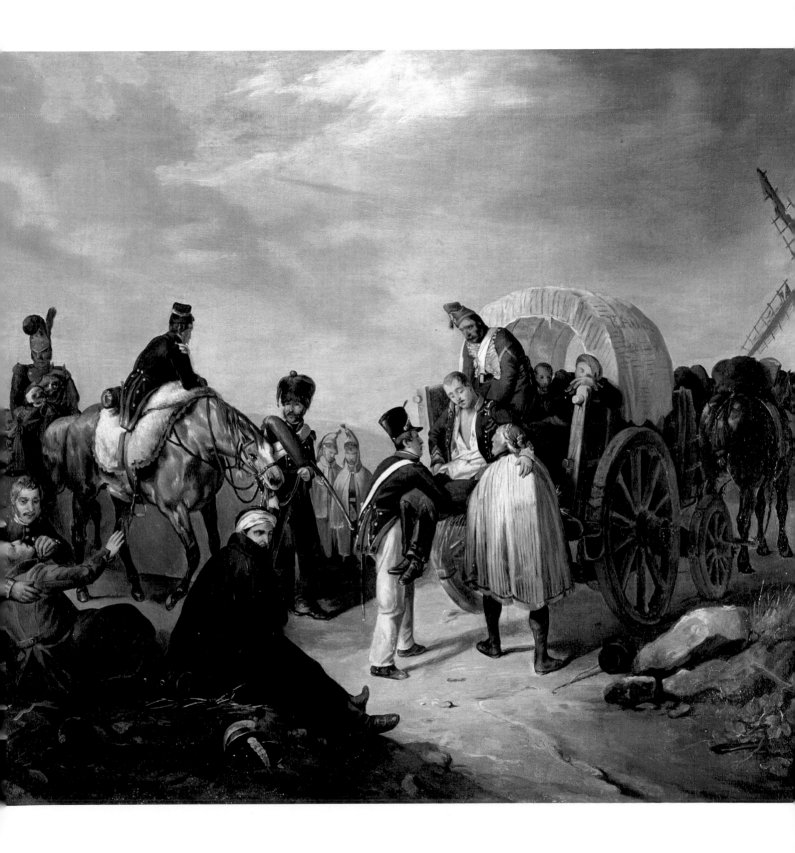

THE CRIMEAN WAR (1853–1856)

Fought between Russia on one side and an alliance of Britain, France, and the Ottoman Empire on the other, the Crimean War created unprecedented problems for the military because it used "modern" technology, causing injuries on a scale never seen before. It was also fought across a hostile terrain where there was a risk of epidemic diseases such as typhoid. Most of the battles took place on the Crimean peninsula, and the poor treatment of wounded and sick soldiers was brought to the attention of the British public by war correspondents, particularly those writing for *The Times*. This resulted in a demand for nursing care, and led to Florence Nightingale's expedition. The Crimean War was the first conflict in which nursing care was offered to troops by professional trained nurses rather than by orderlies and camp-followers.

Florence Nightingale (1820–1910)

One of the most famous women of modern times, Florence Nightingale was a rare individual—a woman who was admired, even revered, in her own time. Indeed, she used the adulation of her contemporaries quite deliberately to push through the many reforms she envisioned—including the development of a secular (nonsectarian) training school for nurses.

Florence was born in the Italian city of Florence on May 12, 1820, into an affluent and well-educated family. Her parents were on an extended honeymoon tour of Europe at the time, and her sister, Parthenope, had been born in Athens the year before. Like all genteel women of her generation, Florence was educated at home, largely by her highly intellectual father. Her mother's family had strong Unitarian connections and had been closely involved in projects for social reform, such as the abolition of the slave trade. As Florence grew up, therefore, she was accustomed to meeting and conversing with intelligent, high-ranking, and often politically powerful individuals, whose radical, reforming views she came to share.

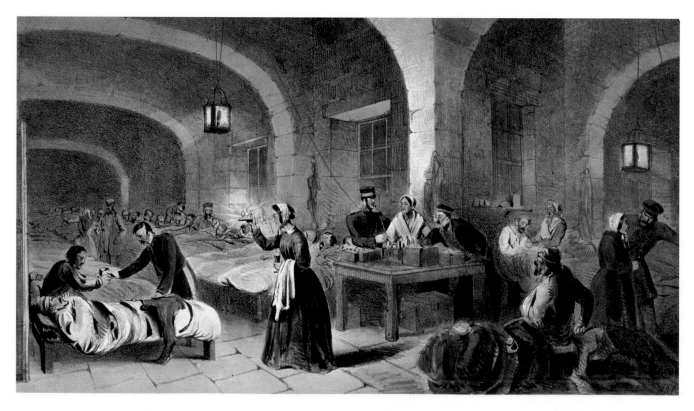

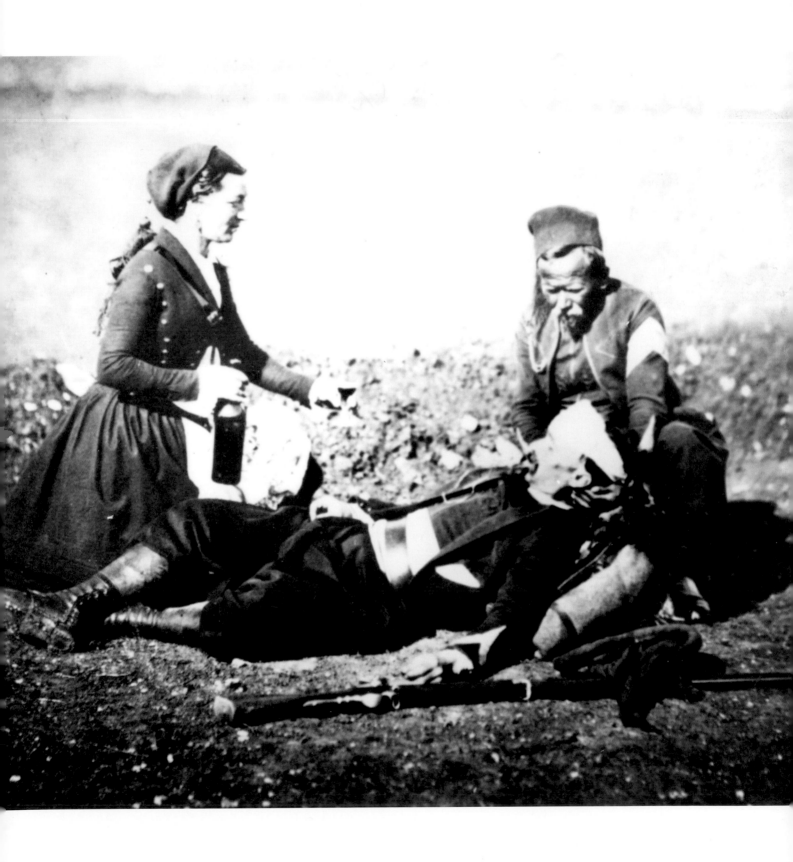

At the age of sixteen Florence had a visionary experience, which she believed was a call from God to give her life to the service of others. Over the next four years, she became more and more certain that the work to which she had been called was nursing. Unfortunately, by the early nineteenth century nursing had long been viewed as an occupation suitable only for women of low social class and very poor reputation. In the 1830s, it was highly unusual for a young genteel girl to want to do nursing work, and it is not surprising that her parents opposed her at first. For many years she struggled against the prejudices of her family, and these years were intensely difficult ones.

The turning point came in 1850, when Florence was able to spend two weeks visiting the Kaiserswerth Institution in Germany (see page 37). Although she was quite critical of the nursing training that took place there, Florence was impressed by the way the institution was run, and was encouraged in her determination to develop nursing in Britain. Three years later, she was offered her first position as a nurse when she became Superintendent of the Establishment for Gentlewomen during Illness in London, England. Before taking up the post, she spent time in several Paris hospitals, where she observed the nursing care offered by Augustinian and other French nursing sisters and worked under the supervision of the Sisters of Charity at the Maison de la Providence.

Florence had only been at the Establishment for Gentlewomen for about seventeen months when the call came from her old friends Sidney and Elizabeth Herbert to lead a party of nurses to the Crimea. British troops fighting alongside the French against the Russians were dying in their thousands, not just from their battle injuries but also from the enteric diseases that were rife in the overcrowded Scutari barracks hospital in Turkey. It became clear that the nursing care offered to these desperately ill and wounded men was inadequate, particularly when compared with the expert care offered by French and Russian sisterhoods. The scandal was reported in *The Times* newspaper, and caused a great furore in Britain. The government was forced to respond, and Herbert, as Secretary of State for War, called upon Florence to help.

The nurses Florence took with her to Turkey included members of the Sellonite and St John's Sisterhoods (see page 40), Catholic nuns from the Bermondsey Convent in East London, experienced working-class hospital nurses, and lady nurses like herself. At first the Chief Medical Officer, Dr John Hall, would not allow them to practice and the nurses were reduced to merely preparing dressings and cleaning their quarters. Eventually, however, the arrival of large contingents of wounded from Sebastopol and other battles forced the medical staff to call on the help of Florence's nurses. Their work at Scutari set the seal on Florence's fame.

When Florence fell ill with "Crimean fever" (probably the disease brucellosis) in 1856, the press reported daily on her progress, and her recovery was a cause for national celebration. However, that recovery was never really complete and Florence was to undergo a serious relapse in 1857 from which she never really recovered. She was to experience illness, debility, and pain for the rest of her life.

Right:
Florence Nightingale;
Frances Parthenope,
Lady Verney (c.1836) by
William White. In this
portrait of the Nightingale
sisters as young girls,
Florence is seated, while her
sister Parthenope stands to
her left holding a book.

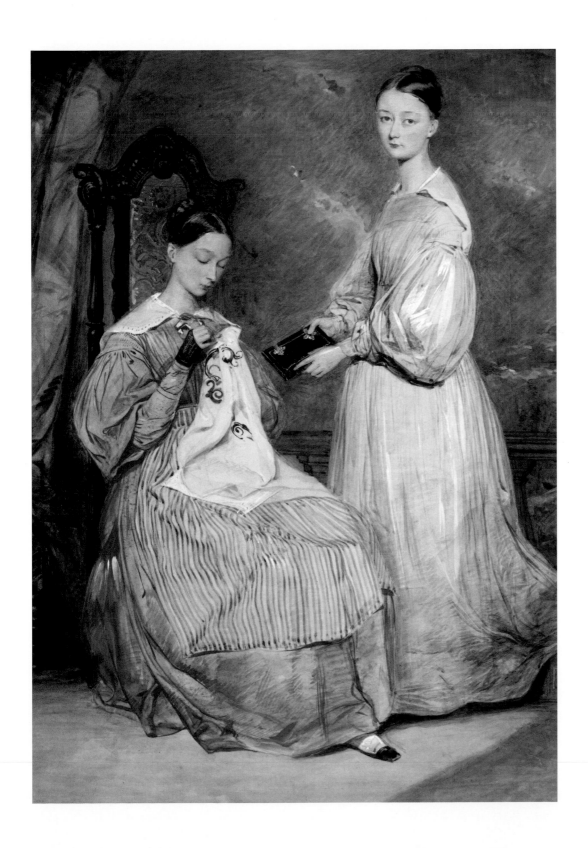

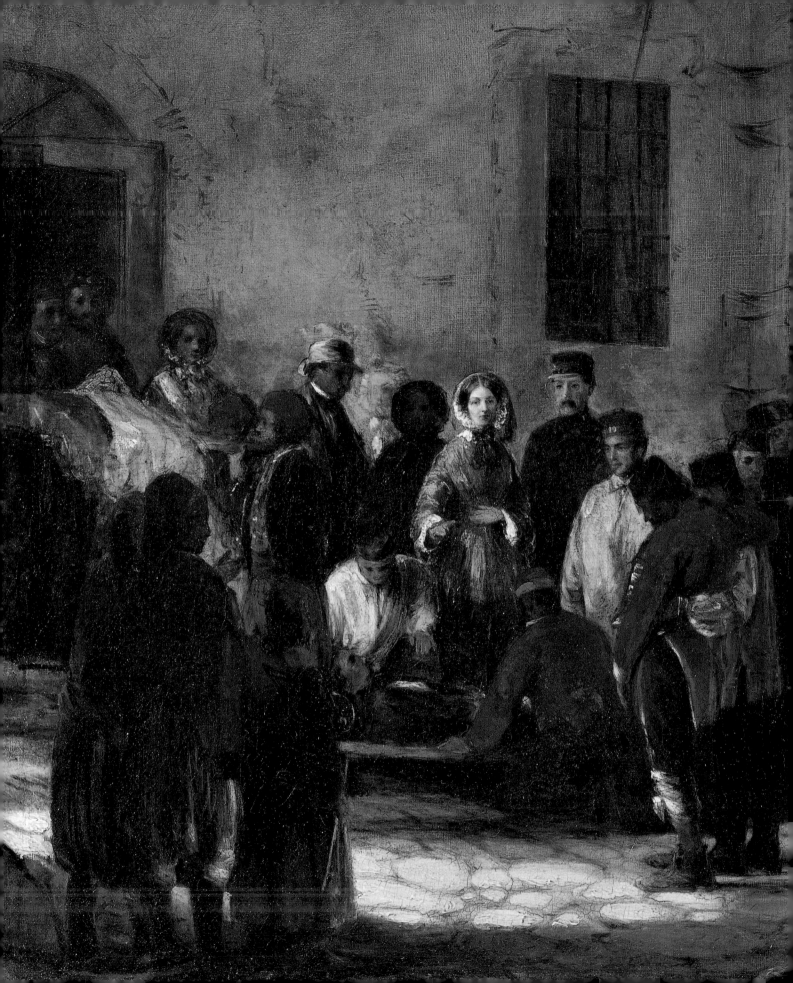

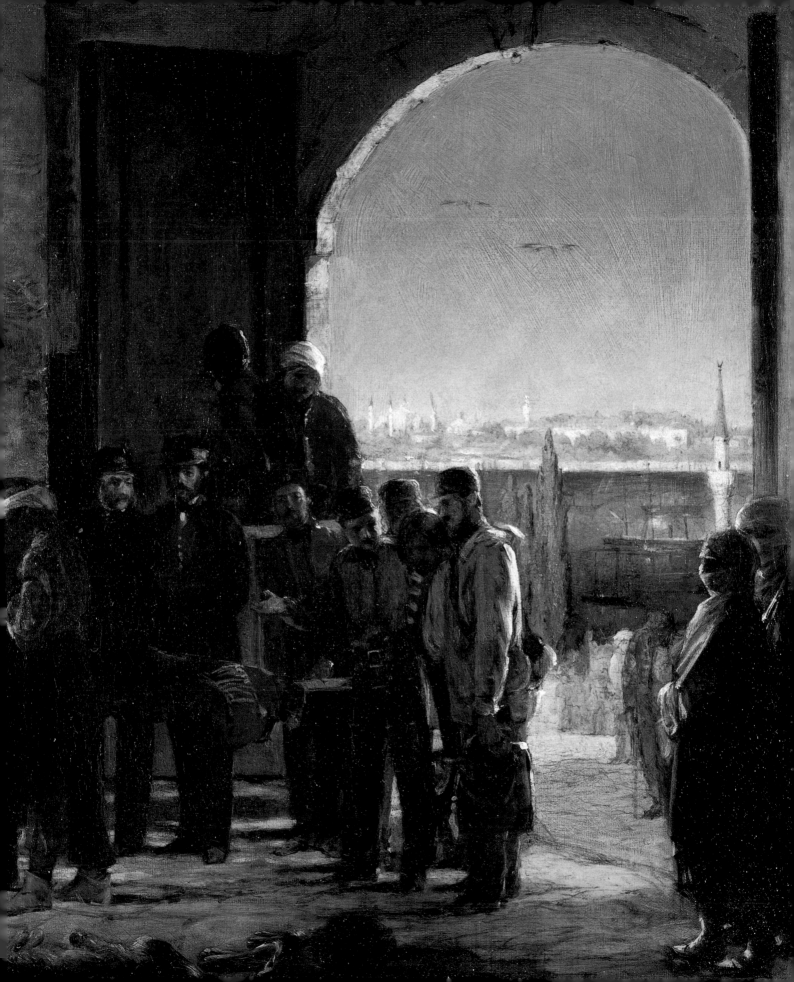

Previous pages:
Florence Nightingale
Receiving the Wounded at
Scutari *(1856) by Jerry
Barrett. Florence stands
illuminated in the center,
flanked by the nursing nun
Mary Clare Moore (on her
right) and Selena Bracebridge
(on her left). The soldier in the
foreground is tended by nurse
Eliza Roberts.*

Right:
*Florence Nightingale, shown
in her later years.*

Opposite:
*Jamaican-born Mary
Seacole traveled alone to the
Crimea to work as a
"nurse and doctress."*

Ironically, the arrival of Florence's party did not lead to a reduced mortality rate at the Scutari barracks hospital. Indeed, when Florence studied the statistics later with Dr John Sutherland, a member of the Sanitary Commission to the East, she was dismayed to discover that mortality rates had actually risen during her time there. Florence realized this was probably due to poor sanitary conditions. Determined that these should never recur, she devoted much of her time to sanitary reform, including a huge project to promote the reform of the Army Medical Services in Britain through her work for the Royal Commission on the Health of the Army. She also worked tirelessly to improve sanitary conditions in India.

As a result of her popularity a national appeal for nursing funds was launched in August 1855 and raised £44,039, a sum that became known as the Nightingale Fund. The money was offered to Florence to be used to found a training school for nurses. Through the development of this training school at St Thomas's Hospital, London, her work on the development of District Nursing, and her writings such as *Notes on Nursing* (published in 1859/60), Florence came to have a lasting influence on the nursing profession.

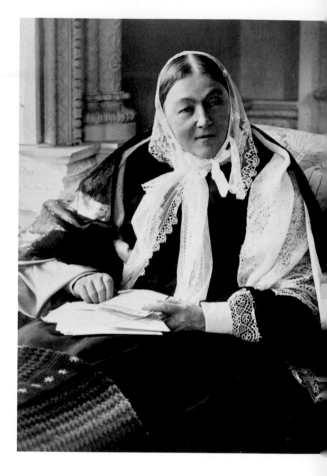

"*One's feelings waste themselves in words; they ought all to be distilled into actions . . . which bring results.*"

Florence Nightingale

Letter to a friend, quoted in The Life of Florence Nightingale *by Edward Tyas Cook (1913)*

Mary Seacole (1805–1881)

Born Mary Jane Grant in Kingston, Jamaica, Mary Seacole traveled to the Crimea to care for the injured and dying on the battlefields. Her mother was a Creole and her father a Scottish army officer. Mary's application to join the second party of British nurses leaving for the Crimea in late 1854 was rejected—on account of her color, she believed. She therefore went to the Crimea as an independent "nurse and doctress," where she established a hotel at Spring Hill (near Balaclava) for soldiers, and successfully treated cases of dysentery with Caribbean herbal remedies. Her memoir, *The Wonderful Adventures of Mrs Seacole in Many Lands*, published in 1857, stands as one of the liveliest and most intriguing autobiographies of its day.

Mary Clare Moore (1814–1874)

One of the most successful Catholic nursing nuns of her time, Mary Clare Moore became Mother Superior of the newly founded convent of the Sisters of Mercy, Bermondsey, in South London, in 1839. This was the first convent to be established in Britain since the Catholic Emancipation Act of 1829 had made such foundations legal for the first time since the Reformation. Although very young and inexperienced, Mary was considered by Catherine McAuley, the founder of the Sisters of Mercy in Ireland, to be the best candidate for the job. McAuley was not mistaken. Mary ran the controversial London convent with grace and wisdom. She also led a contingent of the most effective nurses to join Florence Nightingale in the Crimea, and became one of Florence's lifelong friends and confidantes. Alongside her in the Crimea were two of her most effective colleagues, Mary Stanislaus Jones and Mary Gonzaga. Florence called Gonzaga "my Cardinal" and made her the head of Scutari's General Hospital.

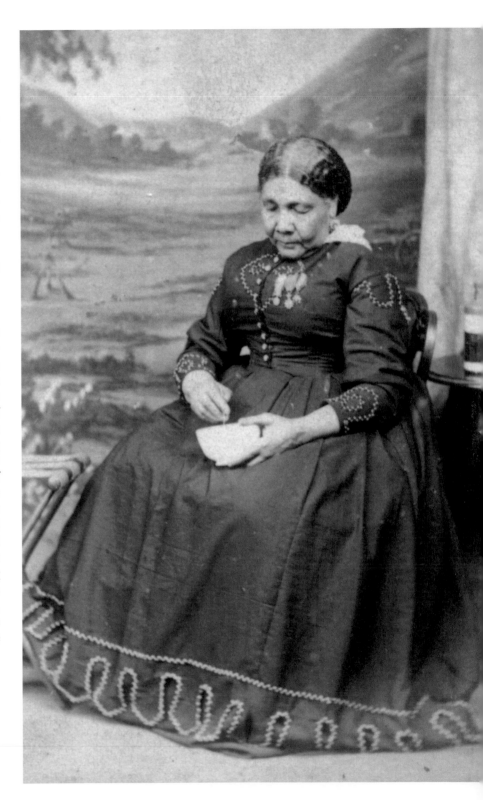

THE AMERICAN CIVIL WAR
(1861–1865)

Like any civil war, the American Civil War found
people unprepared, both for the conflict itself and
for the havoc it would create. At first the
government sought the help of Catholic Sisters,
who already ran a number of hospitals and were
clearly the most skilled individuals to care for the
wounded. Important work was undertaken by
hundreds of nursing sisters under the leadership of
indomitable women such as Mother Gonzaga of the
Satterlee Hospital, Philadelphia, and Mother
Angela of the Mound City Hospital, Illinois.
But their numbers were insufficient, and the
government established a volunteer nursing service
under Dorothea Dix, who was appointed Superintendent of Female Nurses for the Army.

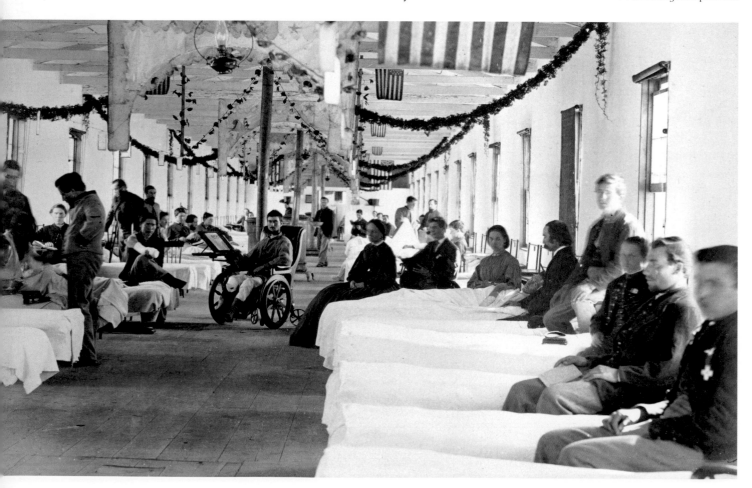

Dorothea Dix (1802–1887)

A remarkable woman, Dorothea Dix had a strength of character that was clearly molded by her early experiences. She had a very difficult childhood, and at the age of twelve ran away from home—and from her alcoholic, abusive father—to live with her grandmother. In her thirties, she undertook important work as a reformer of mental hospitals. Although Dorothea struggled to develop the nursing services, and often found herself in conflict with her army medical colleagues, she made a name for herself by her insistence that her nurses offer the same standard of care to both Unionist and Confederate wounded.

Volunteer Training

In all, more than 2,000 women served as volunteer nurses during the civil war. Many did extraordinary work. Some also showed amazing courage, such as the famous "Mother Bickerdyke," who attended the wounded of nineteen battles and went out onto battlefields at night with a lantern, searching among the dead for wounded men who had been missed by stretcher-bearers.

Temporary hospitals were established in country houses, tents, and public buildings, including the Capitol at Washington, where patients were nursed in the Senate and the Rotunda. Steamers on the Mississippi were converted into hospital ships. In these hospitals the work of caring for patients was shared by nursing sisters, male orderlies, and female volunteers, who dressed wounds, gave medicines and diets, and offered care and comfort. Yet the lack of an organized nursing service meant that the wounded were lucky if they found their way to a hospital where effective care was offered. Many were laid in temporary shelters with no nurses to care for them and only a few surgeons to treat their wounds. Shortages of supplies meant that many patients went without clean clothes, and the lack of expert attention to wounds meant that gangrene was common. In many ways, the example of their suffering illustrates the vital importance of providing expert nursing in times of war.

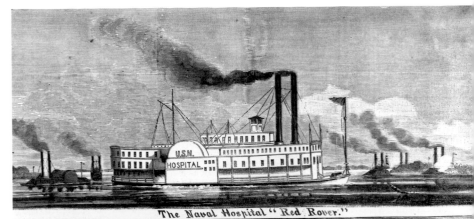

The Naval Hospital "Red Rover."

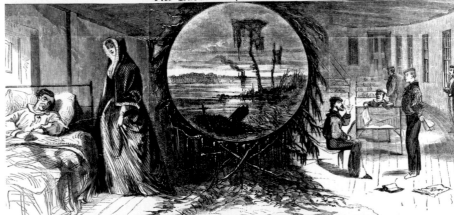

"The Sister."　　　Convalescent Ward.

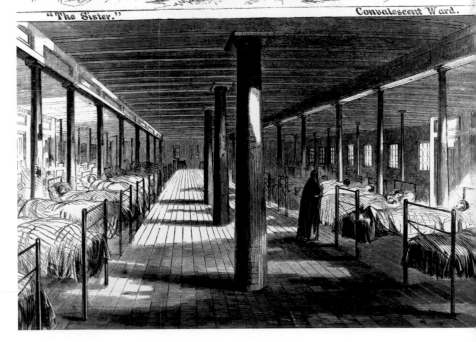

Walt Whitman (1819–1892)

The poet Walt Whitman—author of the controversial epic poem, *Leaves of Grass*—served as a volunteer nurse in the Union Army hospitals in Washington D.C. He traveled from his home in New York to search for his brother George, who had been reported wounded. Finding his brother alive and well, he decided to offer his services as a volunteer-nurse, obtaining a job as a part-time clerk in the army paymaster's office to support himself while he did this work. He later wrote of his experiences in *Memoranda During the War*, in which he bore witness to the horrific nature of war-injury and disease.

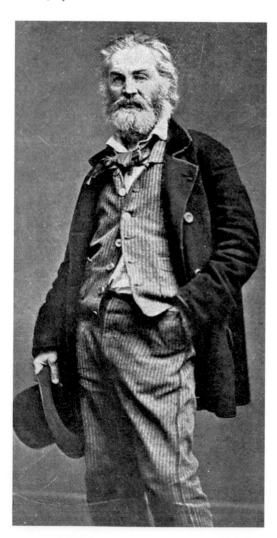

Clara Barton (1821–1912)

Born Clarissa Harlowe Barton on December 25, 1821, Clara Barton was the fifth child of farmers Sarah and Stephen Barton, who ran a sawmill in Oxford, Massachusetts. She worked as a schoolteacher and then as a clerk in Washington D.C. When war broke out she volunteered to do nursing work, and was eventually made Superintendent of Nurses for the Army of the James. Courageous in the extreme, she joined troop movements so that she could be where the fighting was at its most fierce, and worked close to the front lines, dodging bullets to offer care to the wounded. In August 1862, immediately after the Second Battle of Bull Run, she found herself caring for 3,000 wounded men with only one other nurse, no equipment, and pails of water. In September of the same year, Clara made her way to the Battle of Antietam and assisted at surgical operations, administering chloroform to patients at dressing stations close to the front line. She came to be known as the Angel of the Battlefield.

In March 1865, Abraham Lincoln made Clara Supervisor of the government office of missing soldiers. She and her team located the burial places of 22,000 men and published their names and the locations of their graves.

In 1870, she traveled to the battlefields of the Franco-Prussian War. While in Europe, she learned of the work of the International Committee of the Red Cross and became determined to found a Red Cross Association in the USA. Clara died of pneumonia in 1912, having devoted her life to the care of sick and wounded soldiers.

Right:

American poet Walt Whitman—a classic example of a civilian who volunteered to do nursing work during the Civil War. He worked as an orderly in various Union Army hospitals in Washington D.C.

Opposite:

Clara Barton's work during the American Civil War provided the inspiration for her later foundation of the American Red Cross Association.

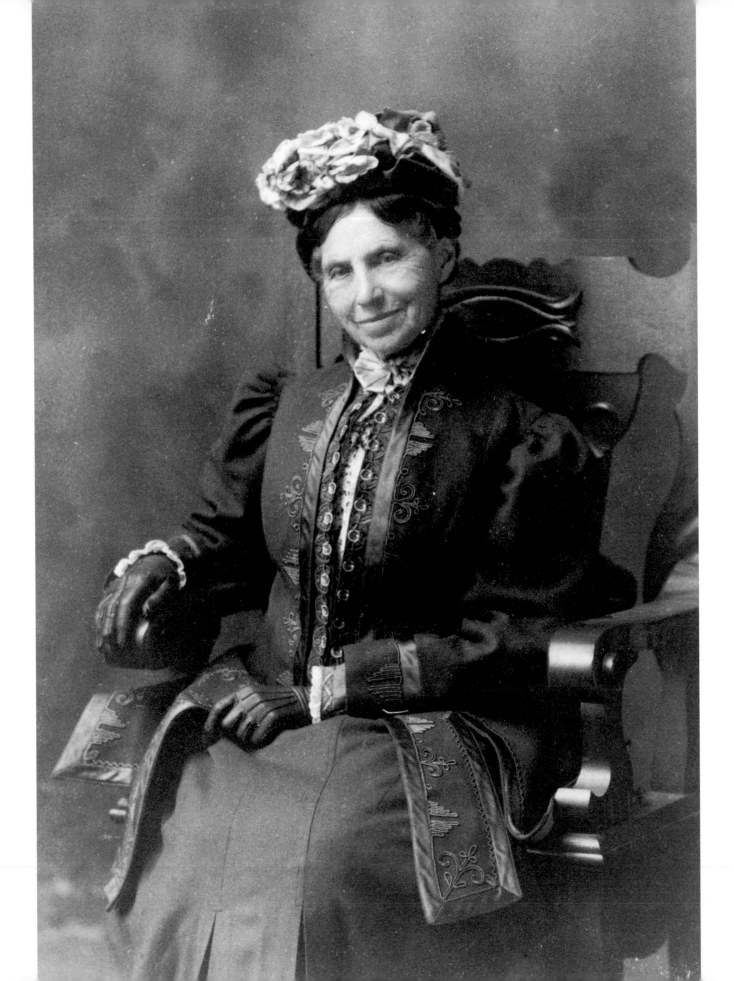

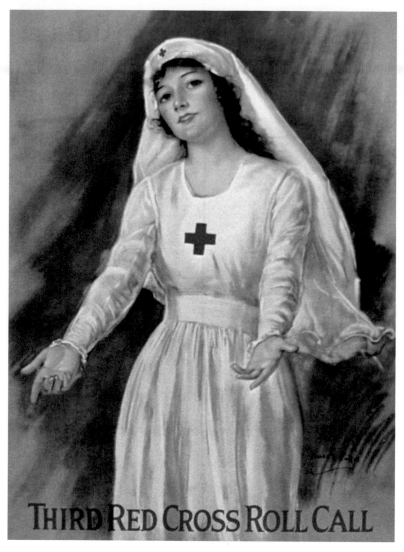

THIRD RED CROSS ROLL CALL

Above:

*Red Cross Associations
throughout the world used
emotive advertising in order
to recruit nurses, as shown
in this American First World
War recruitment poster.*

THE RED CROSS

The creation of the International Committee of the Red Cross was largely due to the efforts of the Swiss social activist, Henri Dunant. After visiting the battlefield of Solferino, Italy, in 1859, Dunant put together a plan by which individual societies would be created in all nations to undertake the work of caring for the wounded in wartime. A central committee would coordinate their efforts. Dunant's plans were agreed at an international conference that was held in Geneva, Switzerland, in 1863. In 1864, a more formal diplomatic agreement was drawn up by fourteen nations, which became known as the Geneva Convention—eventually to be recognized as part of international law.

The Red Cross was to become a movement that would provide relief to those afflicted by natural disaster as well as by warfare. In some European nations, the Red Cross nurse became a familiar figure, and the Red Cross provided important training programs for nurses.

The Red Cross Association of the United States of America was established as a result of a campaign by Clara Barton, and was given official and political recognition in 1882. The committee provided important aid and support through a number of terrible natural disasters, such as the Michigan forest fires of 1881, the Mississippi floods of 1882–83, the Texas famine of 1885, and the Florida yellow fever epidemic of 1888. Its members also did important work during the 1898 Spanish-American War. The first official Red Cross Nursing Service in the USA was established in 1909. Its central committee consisted of ten nurses, and was chaired by Jane Delano, who did important work during the First World War.

Jane Delano (1862–1919)

An influential figure in American nursing, Jane Delano helped develop the nursing services of the USA, and gave military nursing much of its character. She graduated from Bellevue Hospital in 1886, and was Superintendent of Nurses at Philadelphia's University of Pennsylvania Hospital from 1891 to 1896. For a time, she held the position of Superintendent of the Army Nurse Corps, and then became Chair of the Red Cross Committee of Nurses. She was also, for three years, President of the American Nurses Association. It was largely thanks to Jane Delano that the US Army Nurse Corps and the American Red Cross Nursing Service worked so closely together and were able to do such important and influential work in Europe during the First World War.

By the end of the nineteenth century, trained, experienced cadres of military nurses were beginning to emerge in Britain and North America. The British had sent a contingent of nurses to the Boer War in South Africa and in the USA the Red Cross was already exerting an important influence in the development of military nursing as a distinct specialism.

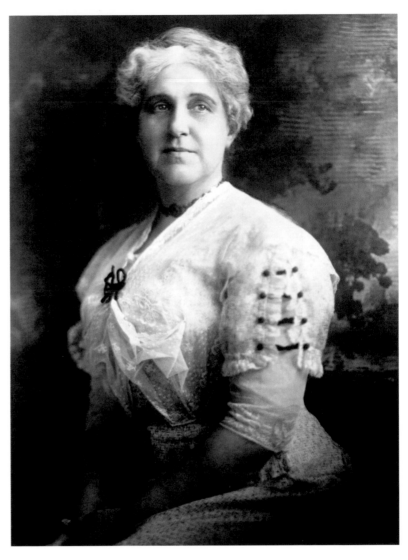

Above:
Jane Delano was Chair of the American Red Cross Committee of Nurses. She played an important role in the development of both civilian and military nursing in the USA.

What is a Nurse?

By the mid-nineteenth century, two classes of nurse were emerging: working-class women who nursed for a living, and philanthropic "ladies" who undertook nursing as a charitable act. In Britain, the latter practiced under the Protestant Nursing Sisterhoods, such as St John's House and the All Saints Sisterhood, both in London. After 1860, secular nursing schools proliferated rapidly, guided by the example of the Nightingale Training School. But before this very few nurses had any formal training. What little there was depended on the efforts of strong-minded individuals.

A NURSE'S EXPERIENCE

We know something of the lives of women who trained in sisterhoods because of a memoir left by one of the sisters, who was known as Sister Eva. After her training, Eva worked in a London hospital, and as a private-duty nurse. She wrote vividly of her experiences.

Sister Eva

There is no information about how old Sister Eva was when she entered nursing, but she describes herself as naïve and inexperienced. She found that joining her sisterhood was similar to entering a convent: she slept on a thin straw mattress, and had only one drawer for all her possessions. Her training was tough, and involved a lot of domestic chores, alongside the development of nursing skills.

One of Eva's more dramatic stories is the tale of her first-ever private duty call, to a woman suffering from both cancer and delirium tremens. Eva found her way through the dark, damp alleyways of the London slums until she arrived at a "poor tumble-down cottage." Her patient was a tall, "bloated" woman with "wild, glaring eyes," who was clearly experiencing a dangerous hallucination. The moment she saw Eva, she attacked her, pushed her to the ground, and dragged her across the room by her hair. At the moment when she was about to be stamped to death by her assailant, Eva gathered her wits and shouted "Don't do that," in what she hoped was a tone of authority. The patient's anger subsided, and she allowed herself to be put to bed. She then lapsed into a coma from which she never recovered. Eva remained with her until she died.

Another of Eva's reminiscences tells of a 29-year-old patient who had suffered a long illness and was not expected to recover. His wife and the nurse were at his bedside when the patient stirred, complained of the dark, and asked for "more air." He seemed to be dying. He asked his wife and then the nurse to kiss him. The wife urged Eva to do as he asked and she "drew near and kissed his cold, damp forehead."

Within hours, the patient amazed his carers by beginning to recover, and after six weeks, was convalescing. Eva recalled his banter:

" 'Well Nellie,' he said, turning to his wife with a merry twinkle in his eyes, the day before I left him, 'Sister did kiss me once, and I thought it so sweet that I determined to live and have another, and here she refuses to give it to me; I think that I deserve one.' I left it an open question, for he certainly never had a second."

Sister Eva's apparently simple stories, presented as Victorian morality tales, mask the complexity of the nursing work she was doing. At the end of her book, *Scenes in the Life of a Nurse (1890)*, she comments on this, hinting also that she has left out some details in order to protect the sensibilities of the reader.

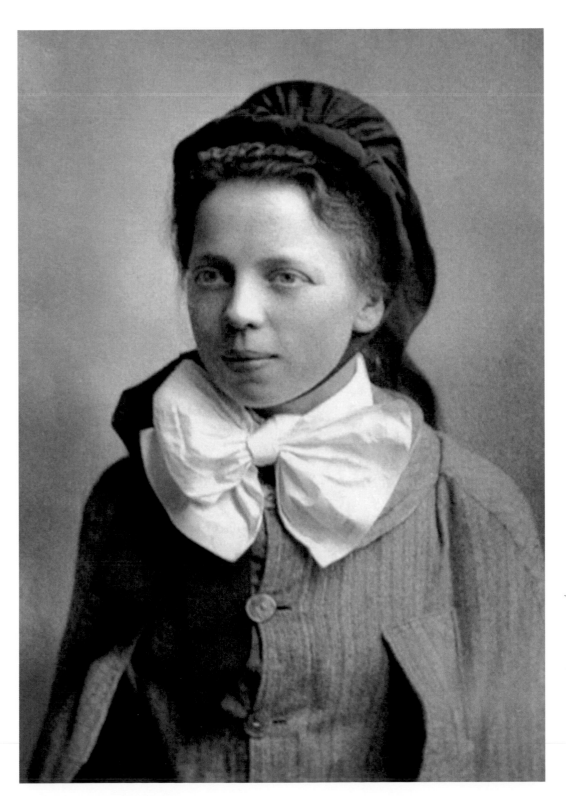

Left:
*Portrait of Sister Eva,
taken from the
frontispiece to her book,*
Scenes in the Life of a
Nurse *(1890). This
memoir provides an image
of a rather "prim and
proper" nurse who wears
her respectability like a
cloak. It also gives a sense
of the depth of her know-
ledge of human nature—
right down to its darkest
recesses—and of how
closely and secretly she
holds that knowledge.*

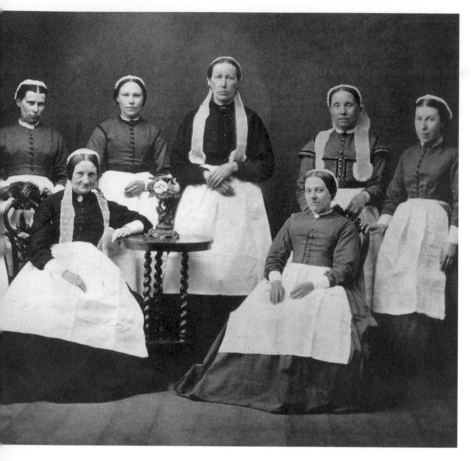

Above:

*The nineteenth century
saw the emergence of a
two-tier nursing
profession, as institutions
retained their older
working-class nurses
while taking on
newer "lady nurses."
This photograph shows
a group comprising
both types of nurse.*

THE LATE NINETEENTH CENTURY

As the nineteenth century progressed, educated nurses continued to hide many of the realities of nursing work, and by the 1870s two types of nurse seemed to exist. First, there were the new lady nurses, such as Florence Nightingale, who were widely admired—by this time, society had identified them as its heroines and had effectively placed them on a pedestal. There were also many working-class nurses, whose presence in hospital wards was essential to the performance of good nursing care. In contrast to the adulation society heaped upon ladies such as Florence Nightingale, it appeared to feel something like contempt for working women. Yet these lower-class nurses, who were largely anonymous, did much of the hard work that took place in hospital wards, and their work merged into the domestic labor of the ward maids.

The ambivalence with which society viewed the "dirty work" associated with nursing was resolved by the apparent emergence of this two-tier system, in which lower-class nurses and ward maids were responsible for cleanliness while the lady-nurses supervised them and performed more "technical" or "scientific" work, such as administering medications or carrying out complex wound-dressings. Yet the secret that only the lady nurses knew was that they too knew how to do "dirty work" with their own hands. Some did take on a purely supervisory role once trained, yet as probationers they had learned their art by performing hands-on nursing care.

To protect their reputations, lady nurses presented themselves as so pure in their starched dresses and white caps that it was difficult for their contemporaries to believe that they had actually touched a patient. Nevertheless, however much they might project an image of themselves as somehow removed from the dirt and squalor of illness, even lady nurses recognized that providing a clean sickroom and caring for the bodies of their patients was an essential part of nursing. From Nightingale onward, nurses had attempted to resolve this split in their working practice. What most really wanted was a unified nursing profession—one whose members were expert in providing both the comfort their patients needed and the technical treatments dictated by the new medical and surgical discoveries. They battled with a social perception that saw some elements of nursing care as "simple" or "basic" and others as "complex," arguing that the nursing care of a patient was a complete whole that could not be split into two. But for the sake of survival they continued to entertain the fiction that nursing was a two-tier profession.

Dressing suppurating and foul-smelling wounds and washing bodies bathed in the sweat of fever were actions that had been valued as "self-sacrificing" by the religious societies of the medieval and early modern worlds. But in an increasingly secular society, self-sacrifice was beginning to lose its romance, and nurses were searching for a more "modern" way of gaining support. One of their approaches was to embrace the technologies of medical science. Another, in those belligerent times, was to play a heroic role on the battlefield. Yet another was to create a professional elite that would fight for status and recognition. In the nineteenth century, it seemed as if nursing could only become great if it also fragmented itself.

Right:
Staff of the Edinburgh Royal Infirmary, Scotland, at the turn of the century.

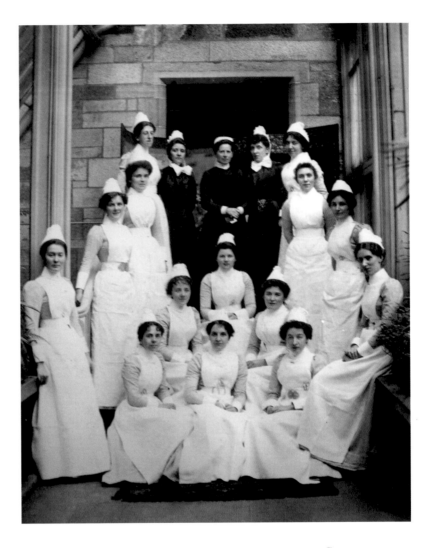

"*The amount of relief and comfort experienced by [the] sick after the skin has been washed and dried, is one of the commonest observations made at a sick bed …They are, in fact, nothing more than a sign that the vital powers have been relieved by removing something that was oppressing them.The nurse, therefore, must never put off attending to the personal cleanliness of her patient.*"

Florence Nightingale

Extract from Notes on Nursing *(1859/60)*

POOR LAW NURSING IN BRITAIN

Florence Nightingale had always wanted her work to lead to social reform in Britain. Although she believed that nurses must be of impeccable moral fiber, and promoted nursing as a profession for educated gentlewomen, she also saw a role for working-class nurses of good character.

Nightingale's first nursing reforms took place in St Thomas's Hospital, a well-funded "voluntary hospital"—one of the hospitals established by the British upper and middle classes for the poor. However, there were also large numbers of other, less prestigious hospitals in Britain that were known as "poor law" infirmaries. Attached to poor-houses, where only those members of society who were utterly destitute and desperate lived, these hospitals were badly funded—places of squalor and neglect. The nursing was undertaken by pauper inmates, who carried out the work in exchange for their accommodation and food. Nightingale decided that she must reform nursing not only in the well-to-do voluntary hospitals but also in these poor law infirmaries.

Her first experiment was to send Agnes Jones, one of her most able St Thomas's nurses, to the Brownlow Hill Workhouse Infirmary in Liverpool as Lady Superintendent.

Agnes Jones (1832–1868)

Born in Dublin, Ireland, the daughter of a British army officer, Agnes was known for her religious piety, but also for her charm and wit. She found her work in the Brownlow Hill Infirmary grueling and depressing, and wrote in her diary of its "dreariness" and "loneliness." Things were not helped by the fact that the hospital governor, George Carr, claimed authority over the nurses, and interfered with her reforms. But Agnes and her team were eventually accepted and made great improvements to the nursing care offered at the infirmary. Agnes died of typhus fever in February 1868, having worked at Brownlow Hill for almost three years.

Right:

Nineteenth-century sketch of The Brownlow Hill Infirmary, Liverpool, England. A crowd is shown gathering as a man is brought in on a stretcher.

Opposite:

Agnes Jones is often regarded as the first professional poor law nurse. She was one of Florence Nightingale's nurses, and after her death Florence wrote an extended essay devoted to her "martyrdom." It is said to have inspired many nurses to enter nursing.

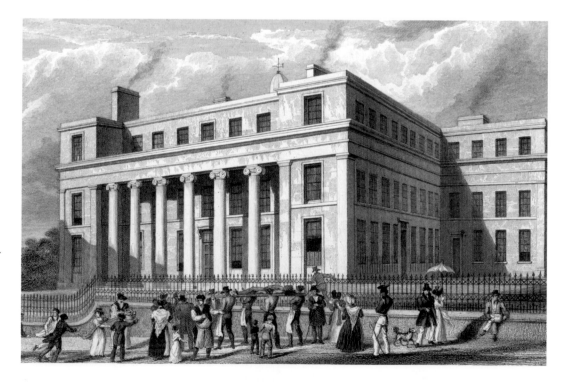

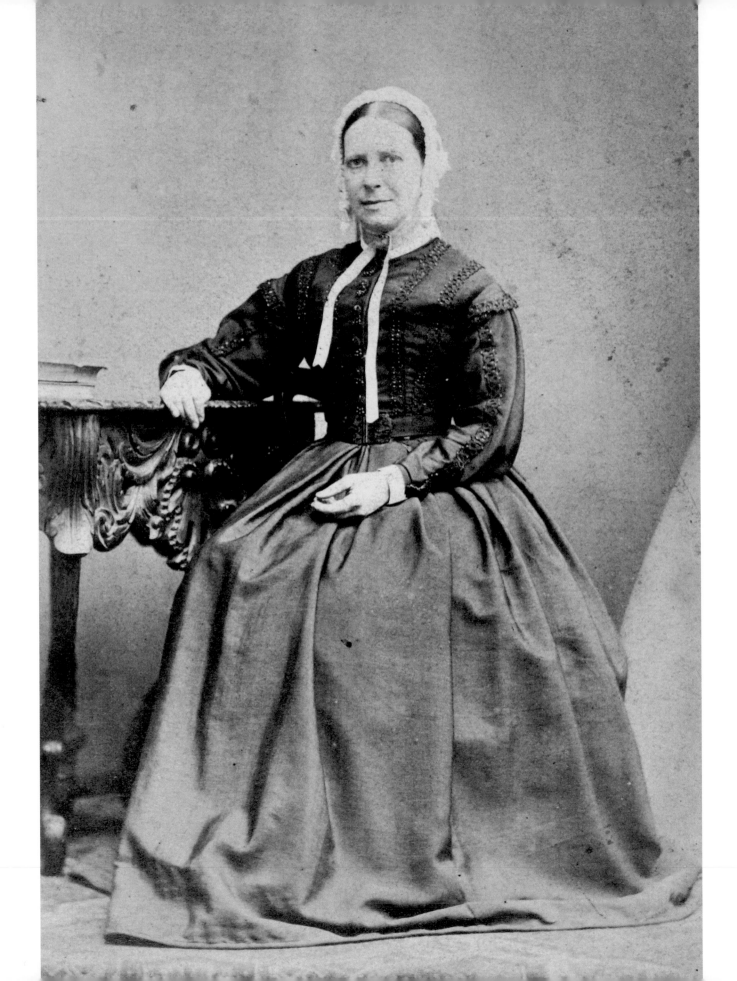

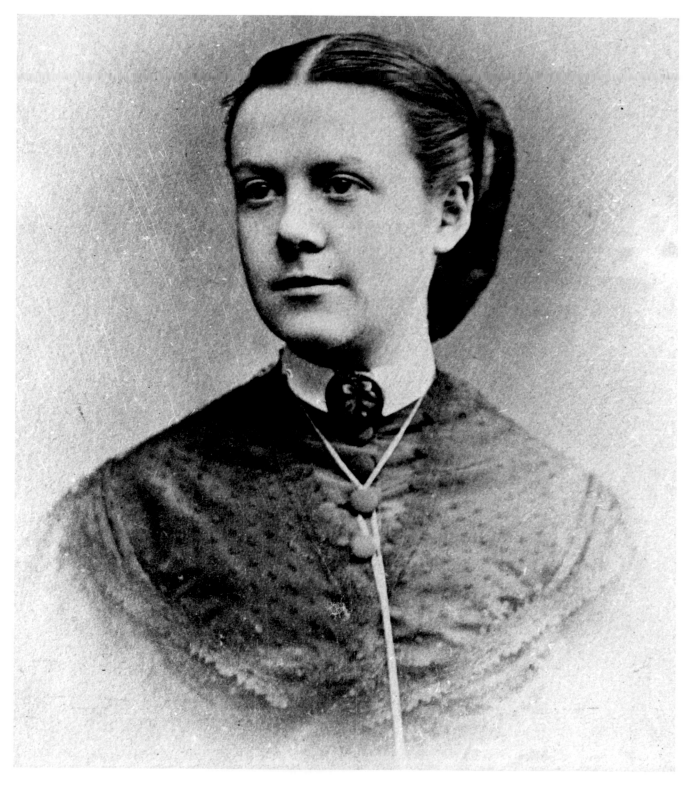

PROFESSIONAL NURSING IN THE USA

The earliest instruction for nurses was offered on a very ad hoc basis by individual hospital doctors who recognized the immense value of the work nurses were doing to improve comfort and reduce mortality rates among patients. Dr Valentine Seaman of the New York Hospital is credited with establishing the first such training at the end of the eighteenth century.

The first formally recognized training schools in the USA were established in 1863. One was at the Woman's Hospital in Philadelphia, from which the first graduate was American Civil War veteran nurse, Harriet Newton Phillips. The other was established by Dr Marie Zakrzewska at the New England Hospital for Women and Children in Boston, Massachusetts. This extraordinary hospital, staffed entirely by women, was granted a charter in 1863, which included the formal recognition of its nurses' training school.

In 1872 the hospital took on a new director, Dr Susan Dimock, and moved into new premises at Roxbury. Susan took the opportunity to establish the nursing school on a firmer footing. Many of its methods came to be based on ideas she had gained in Europe, where she had visited, among other places, the Kaiserswerth Institution in Germany (see page 37).

The New England Hospital for Women and Children struggled for survival at first. Because all of its doctors were women, it was looked down upon by the medical establishment of the day. Its foundation of a nurse training school was part of its battle for survival, and it owed much to the nurses' hard work and enthusiasm.

One of the first five students to graduate from the school was Linda Richards, who became a celebrated figure in American nursing.

Linda Richards (1841–1930)

The youngest of the three daughters of a minister, Linda was born Malinda Ann Judson Richards in 1841. Both her parents died of tuberculosis, her father in 1845 and her mother in 1854. The thirteen-year-old Linda nursed her mother through her final illness. In 1860 she became engaged to George Poole, who soon afterward went to fight in the American Civil War. He was severely injured in 1865, and Linda nursed him until his death in 1869. Linda's experiences of the suffering of those closest to her inspired her to learn more about nursing. She took a job as a nurse at the Boston City Hospital, but found there was no real training there. After only three months' experience, she was offered the position of Head Nurse but declined, because it seemed wrong to her that the nurses at the hospital were treated as maids. She felt that there must be more to the practice of nursing than she had encountered at the Boston City.

Opposite:

Dr Susan Dimock was Director of the New England Hospital for Women and Children.

Below:

Because she was the first nurse to graduate from the New England Hospital for Women and Children, Linda Richards is often referred to as "America's first trained nurse."

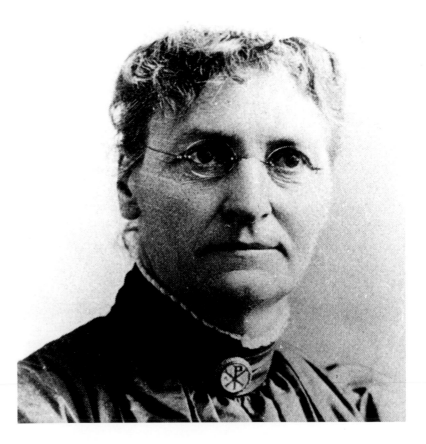

Linda's training at the New England Hospital for Women and Children was difficult. The life was arduous; students received training but were also used as "pairs of hands." Linda later wrote of her training in her well-known book, *Reminiscences*.

The students were given a course of twelve lectures and worked closely with female medical doctors, but there were no examinations. Nurses were not allowed to know the names of the medications they gave to patients. Doctors numbered and labeled these, and then told nurses which to give. Linda is reported to have said later:

"As I look back I wonder that we were as well taught as was really the case and I sometimes feel that we nurses, eager as we were to learn, instructed the physicians nearly as much as they instructed us."

After she had completed her training, Linda became Night Superintendent at the Bellevue Hospital, New York, and then Superintendent of Nurses at the Massachusetts General Hospital. She visited Britain, had meetings with Florence Nightingale, and spent time in King's College Hospital, St Thomas's Hospital, and the Edinburgh Royal Infirmary. She went on to have a highly distinguished career.

In December 1885, she set sail for Japan to establish a nurse training school in Kyoto under the auspices of the American Board of Missions. While there, she organized a two-year training program for nurses, in which lectures were given by medical staff, and American textbooks were used. Linda herself gave classes, with the aid of an interpreter, in which she "translated" the content of medical and surgical lectures to make it relevant to nursing practice.

After her return to the USA, Linda did important pioneering work, establishing institutions for the mentally ill.

"Our days were not eight hours; they were nearer twice eight. We rose at 5.30am and left the wards at 9pm to go to our beds, which were in little rooms between the wards. Each nurse took care of her ward of six patients both day and night. Many a time I have got up nine times in the night; often I did not get to sleep before the next call came."

Linda Richards

Extract from Reminiscences *(2006 edition)*

Right:
By the turn of the century nurse training was incorporating many scientific and technical elements. This photograph shows a group of nurses training in a bacteriology lab.

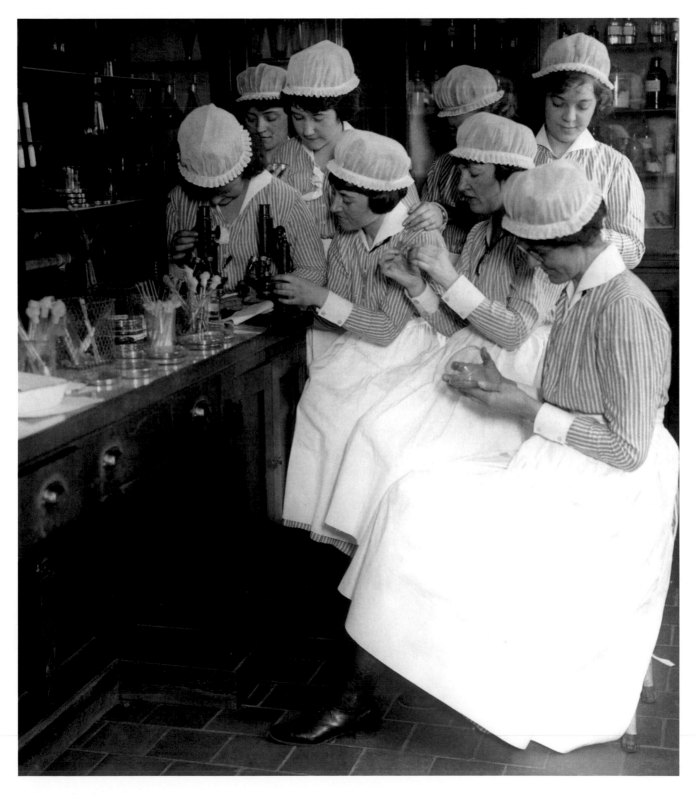

DISTRICT NURSING IN BRITAIN

Nurses are often associated with hospital work, yet some of their most important work has always taken place in patients' own homes. The first experiment in what became known as "district nursing" took place in the British city of Liverpool between 1859 and 1862. The wealthy philanthropist William Rathbone hired a nurse, Mary Robinson, to care for his wife, who was dying of tuberculosis. He was so impressed with her work that he asked her to continue working for him, visiting the sick in the poorest Liverpool households. Eventually, with the help and advice of Florence Nightingale, Rathbone was able to found the Liverpool Training School and Home for Nurses in 1862.

In that same year, the Ladies Sanitary Association in Manchester and Salford developed a visiting service that was to become the forerunner of the British "health visiting" service. This service, which was to become an important focus for public health and welfare work, was to be influential for more than a century. The role of the health visitor was formalized in 1928, when it became impossible for anyone to practice without a certificate from the Royal Sanitary Institute.

A key figure in the development of district nursing in Britain was Florence Lees, who, in 1874, was commissioned by Rathbone to carry out a survey of the work and conditions of district nurses in the London area.

Florence Lees (1840–1922)

Born in Blandford, England, Florence Lees soon decided that she wanted to devote her life to nursing, and at the age of twenty-six, spent four months at the Nightingale Training School as an observer. She then toured Europe, spending time at a number of hospitals and institutions, including the Kaiserswerth in Germany (see page 37). In 1870, she volunteered for service on the German side in the Franco-Prussian War, and was awarded the Order of Merit for her work in military hospitals. But it was for her work in the development of district nursing that she was to become famous.

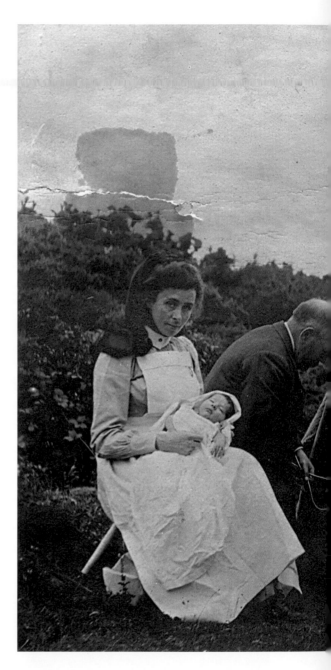

In 1874 Florence wrote a survey of nursing in London, in which she argued strongly for the introduction of a scheme for district nursing there. A year later, she was instrumental in the foundation of the Metropolitan and National Nursing Association for Providing Trained Nurses for the Sick Poor. Its Central Home in Bloomsbury acted

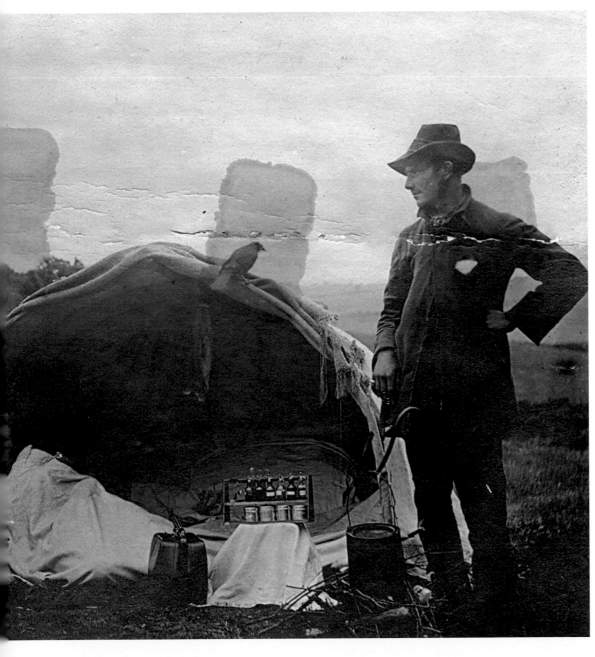

Left:
*Image held by the Royal
College of Nursing UK,
capturing a visit by a nurse
and doctor in a
nineteenth-century rural
setting. In the archive it is
labeled "Nurse Mailer and
local doctor at baby birth
gipsy tent."*

both as an organizing center and as a "nurse's home" for staff. In 1887, Florence was instrumental in persuading Queen Victoria to fund a national organization for district nurses, known as the Queen Victoria Jubilee Institute. Its purpose was declared to be "the nursing of the sick poor in their own homes by trained nurses," and it received its Royal Charter in 1889. In that same year, Florence published her *Guide to District Nurses and Home Nursing*, which had an important influence on the development of District Nursing Associations throughout the country. She died in October 1922, having given much of her life to the development of the nursing profession.

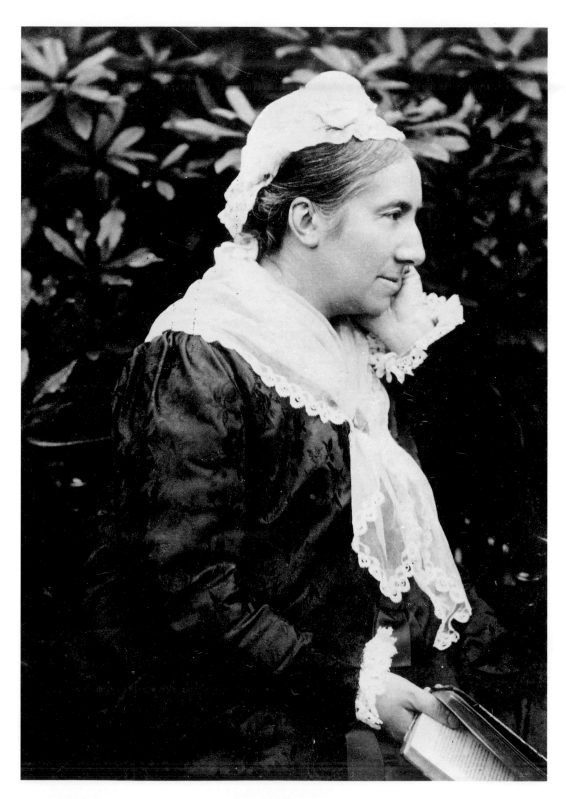

Right:
Elizabeth Malleson, the founder of the Rural Nursing Association.

Elizabeth Malleson (1828–1916)

Born in Chelsea, London, in 1828, Elizabeth Malleson was instrumental in reforming rural nursing in Britain, and founded the Rural Nursing Association. Her parents were highly politically active Unitarians and were often involved in campaigns for social justice which took them away from home. During their frequent absences, Elizabeth took responsibility for the care and education of her younger siblings. She became a teacher in 1852, and spent much of her life campaigning for educational reform. In 1857, she married a successful wine merchant, and in 1882 they moved to the rural English county of Gloucestershire.

At first, far-removed from her reforming activities in London, Elizabeth was unhappy. However, she soon found a new cause when she realized that there was a severe shortage of good nursing care in rural districts. She began by employing a private nurse, known locally as Nurse Mary, in her own parish. However, the experiment lasted only nine months due to a lack of funds. The establishment of the Queen Victoria Jubilee Institute for Nurses (QVJIN) in 1887 gave her the impetus to found the Rural Nurses Association in 1890, which was absorbed into the QVJIN as its "rural arm" in 1897. The establishment of local committees of the Association in rural areas was part of a fascinating movement by which those women who had previously acted as "ladies bountiful," ministering directly to the poor within their own localities, now performed the role of managers and bureaucrats, directing the work of clinical experts.

The nurses employed by the Association had a difficult job. Often covering several miles a day on foot, or by bicycle or donkey-cart, they were said to combine the roles of servant, teacher, and gentlewoman. Most seem to have been very popular with their local communities. Because of a shortage of nurses, gaps in the service were plugged by "village nurse-midwives," with one year's training. They operated ostensibly under the supervision of trained nurses, but in reality had to work very independently in areas where the nearest trained nurse or doctor could be several miles away and impossible to reach quickly in an emergency. The fully trained nurses themselves carried a huge responsibility, dealing with serious injury, illness, and the complications of childbirth, covering thousands of acres and caring for vast, but scattered populations. Unfortunately, they sometimes met with opposition from doctors who were afraid that these highly trained and popular practitioners would rob them of their fee-paying patients and thus threaten their livelihoods.

PUBLIC HEALTH NURSING IN THE USA

In an era when germ theory was just emerging, public health nursing developed as a means to fight infection, poverty, and deprivation. Before the advent of antibiotics, the advice offered by visiting nurses on hygiene, cleanliness, and good diet probably saved more lives than the latest medical technology.

Following the example of the Nightingale Training School in London's St Thomas's Hospital (see page 50), many North American hospitals established their own training schools from the 1870s onward. Students staffed hospital wards, where medical advances were creating a huge need for technically expert practitioners. However, one of the most important spin-offs of this new emphasis on training was the emergence of a cadre of nurses who went on to develop public health practice throughout the USA. In cities, these women countered the negative effects of an Industrial Revolution that had mushroomed out of control, bringing poverty and disease in its wake.

In rural areas nursing work was taken even further. Some of the remotest communities didn't have a doctor or dentist within 100 miles. Here, nurses took on a huge range of practices, pulling teeth, delivering babies, dressing wounds, and offering solace and care to the sick, in addition to bringing the most up-to-date public health knowledge and practice to their communities.

One of the earliest records of visiting nurses dates from 1839, and relates to the work of a Quaker group in Philadelphia, which established an ad hoc service known as the Nurse Society of Philadelphia. Physicians could call upon its nurses, assigning them to individual women from impoverished backgrounds who had recently given birth. By remaining with an individual for several weeks, the nurse could both support the mother and offer advice in the care of her infant, including guidance on sanitation, hygiene, and health. Nurses were paid two and a half dollars per week and were supervised by "lady visitors." By 1850, the Society had employed fifty women, and in that year a "Home and School" was opened. In the 1850s the Society's nurses began to be assigned to medical and surgical, as well as to maternity, cases. In a report of 1867, the Society claimed to have been in continuous existence since 1828, and to be the "First School in America established to Train Women as Nurses."

In the USA, community-based nurses came to be known as visiting nurses, and were administered by Visiting Nurse Associations in many cities. They developed rapidly in the last two decades of the nineteenth century. Philanthropic "lady managers" administered the service provided by working nurses.

Lillian Wald (1867–1940)

Born in Cincinnati, Ohio, on March 10, 1867, Lillian Wald spent her early childhood in Rochester. The daughter of wealthy European immigrants, she attended an English-French boarding school and was said to have been extremely clever from an early age, excelling in both science and the arts. Lillian was present when her sister, Julia, gave birth, and was so impressed by the work of the nurse who attended her that she decided to enter nurse training. She enrolled in the New York Hospital Training School in 1889. After graduating in 1891, she worked for a time at the New York Juvenile Asylum, but hated institutional work. She undertook further study at Women's Medical College in New York City.

Right:
Lillian Wald's early experiences of nursing at the New York Hospital Training School brought her into contact with many patients whose preventable diseases were due to poverty and deprivation. This inspired her to develop a new branch of nursing, which she named "public health nursing."

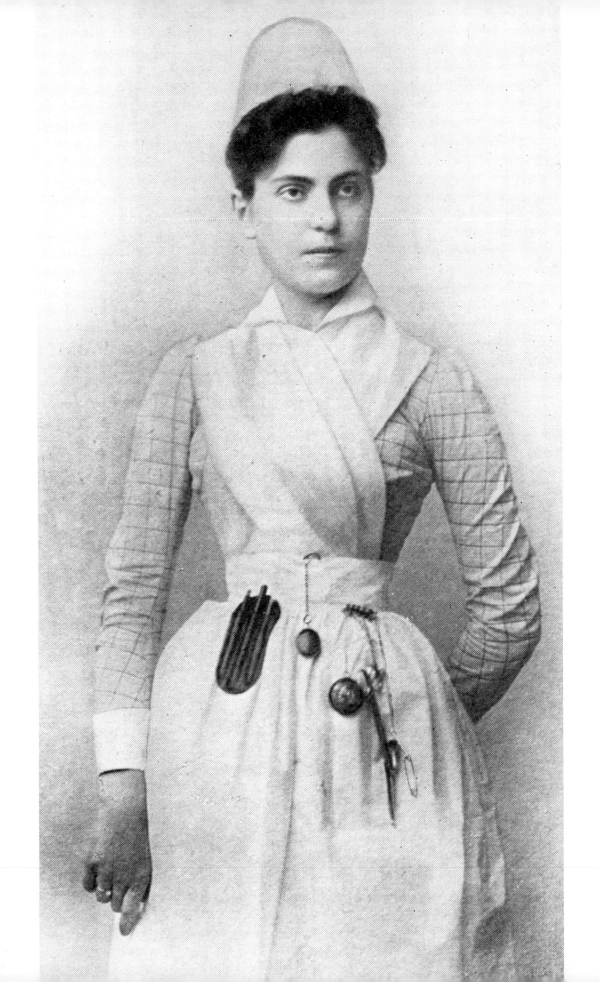

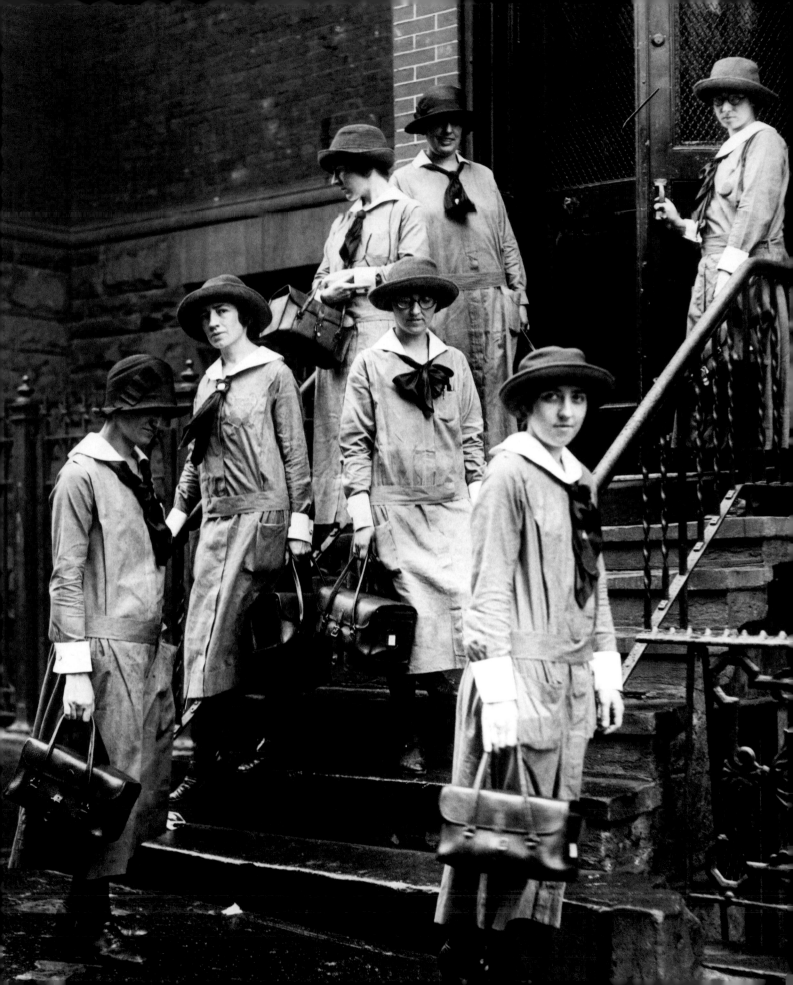

In 1893 Lillian embarked on the most important work of her life: the development of a branch of nursing, which she named "public health nursing." She specialized in the education and care of poor and middle-class New Yorkers, and her work emphasized the importance of empowering people to take control of their own and their families' health. The work for which Lillian is best known was the foundation of the world-famous Henry Street Settlement. Lillian and her friend, Mary Brewster, founded the Visiting Nurses Service in New York City in 1893. In 1895, they moved into Number 265, Henry Street, in New York's Lower East Side (one of the poorest and most deprived parts of the city) and the work of the Settlement was begun. For many years, the building formed the center of operations for the service, and also acted as a nurses' home for some of its members. One of the first things Lillian did was to develop its backyard into a safe play area for neighborhood children. She also established a first-aid room, and her nurses went out to the poorest neighborhoods of the Lower East Side, caring for the sick, and offering health advice and support.

The Settlement grew rapidly, and new branches were opened in Manhattan, the Bronx, and other New York neighborhoods. "Convalescent homes" were established on the Hudson River for those recovering from serious illnesses. Between 1897 and 1900, similar settlements were founded in San Francisco; Los Angeles; Orange, New Jersey; and Richmond, Virginia; and these were clearly inspired by the example of Henry Street.

Lillian Wald's work went much further than the development of a single public nursing service, however. She also campaigned tirelessly to improve the lives of poorer members of society, and to make possible the American dream that all should enjoy "life, liberty, and the pursuit of happiness." It was actually living and working in one of the poorest slums of New York that allowed Lillian to realize just what life was really like for the poor. All too often, the desperate circumstances in which they found themselves made change impossible. She learned firsthand that disease had causes that were beyond the power of the individual to control or escape. She fought for public parks, school nursing services, and free school meals. She campaigned for racial harmony, for the improvement of workers' rights, and for child health and welfare. Lillian was, throughout her life, a great advocate for peace between nations, playing an influential role in the Women's International League for Peace and Freedom. She fought for women's suffrage, partly on the grounds that the presence of women in governments would encourage more pacific international relations.

Lillian had an important influence on the development of nursing education in the USA. She inaugurated a series of lectures at Columbia University Teachers College in 1899, which influenced the later development of the Department of Nursing and Health at the university in 1910. In 1912, Lillian became the first President of the National Organization of Public Health Nurses.

"Never in all the years have we on Henry Street doubted the validity of our belief in the essential dignity of man and the obligations of each generation to do better for the oncoming generation."

Lillian Wald

Quoted on the Jewish Women's Archive web site

Opposite:
Public health nursing developed rapidly during the last decades of the nineteenth century. By the early twentieth century, training for public health practice was based on a clear and recognized body of knowledge. The famous Henry Street Settlement was founded in 1895 by Lillian Wald and Mary Maud Brewster. It provided health care for the poor in the Lower East Side, New York.

THE VICTORIAN ORDER OF NURSES IN CANADA

In the last decade of the nineteenth century, Lady Aberdeen, wife to the Governor-General of Western Canada, began to campaign for the foundation of a district nursing service in Canada. Her campaign was a long and difficult one. It met with opposition from some medical groups, who feared that partially trained nurses, introduced "by the back door," would offer medical treatment in remote areas without supervision. In fact, the service was to consist of doubly qualified nurses, since members had to obtain a diploma in a recognized training school and then gain a further qualification in community work before they could be taken on by the service. A campaign to raise funds for the project was begun and the Victorian Order of Nurses (VON) was founded in February 1897. Toward the end of that year, Charlotte Macleod was made Chief Lady Superintendent, and training homes were established in Montreal and Toronto. On completion of her training, each nurse took a pledge to work for the organization for at least two years either as a district nurse or in a remote cottage hospital.

The Klondyke Expedition

One of the earliest projects of the VON was also one of its most dangerous. In the spring of 1898 a contingent of four district nurses was sent to the Klondyke in the far northern Yukon Territory to serve a population that was suffering as a result of the gold rush. Nurses Powell, Payson, Hanna, and Scott spent several months on the long and difficult journey to Dawson. The District Lady Superintendent of the expedition, "Georgie" Powell, sent a letter home describing their experiences. When they first arrived in the Klondyke, an epidemic of typhoid fever was raging, and men were dying every day. Georgie described how

"on arriving in Dawson with the advance guard of the soldiers, and practically without baggage or nursing provisions, after a march of 150 miles, on August 8th, 1898, I undertook the charge of the Good Samaritan Hospital, entering on my duties as matron, teacher, nurse, and maid of all work on the 11th."

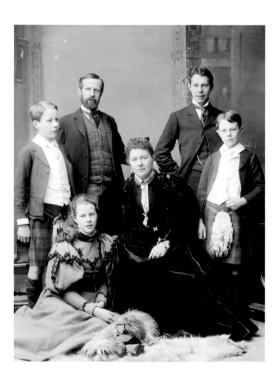

Right:
Lady Aberdeen, wife to the Governor-General of Western Canada, surrounded by her family.

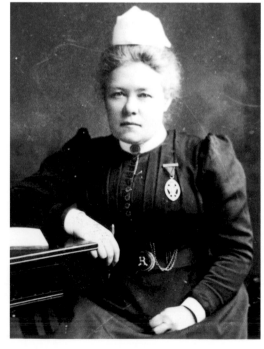

Far right:
Charlotte McLeod, Chief Lady Superintendent of the Victorian Order of Nurses.

The number of typhoid patients increased exponentially after her arrival, yet she and her assistants went out onto the trail to search for men who had collapsed en route to the hospital and bring them to safety. The cases were the most severe she had ever seen. In some, typhoid was combined with pneumonia, malaria, rheumatism, and neuralgia. Mattresses and blankets were in short supply and laundry services were scarce. After four weeks, Georgie herself contracted typhoid and had to hand over the work to one of her colleagues.

Nurse Payson

One of the other nurses, Miss Payson, was sent to Grand Forks Hospital, 12 miles from Dawson. After walking there through snow and slush, she was taken to the hotel, but found herself directed to a room where several men were sleeping. Upon informing the landlord that she had been sent to the wrong room, she was told:

" 'Lor, miss... you will find a row of women on the floor on the other side [the men had beds] and you will find a place all ready for you.' "

When Nurse Payson reached the hospital the next morning, she found that the beds consisted of pole frames with blankets thrown over them. There were no sheets or towels. The nurse's sleeping quarters were a corner of the doctor's office, screened by a curtain where she slept on the floor in her sleeping bag.

The work of the four Klondyke nurses was praised by members of the government, army, and church, and their expedition demonstrated what important work could be done by fully trained nurses in remote outpost areas. Where possible, the nurses worked under medical supervision, but during emergencies, when there was no doctor present, they were forced to act independently and this could increase their scope of practice dramatically. Over the next few decades, the work of the Victorian Order of Nurses expanded rapidly. Many cottage hospitals were built in remote areas, and large numbers of district nurses were taken on to care for scattered and isolated populations.

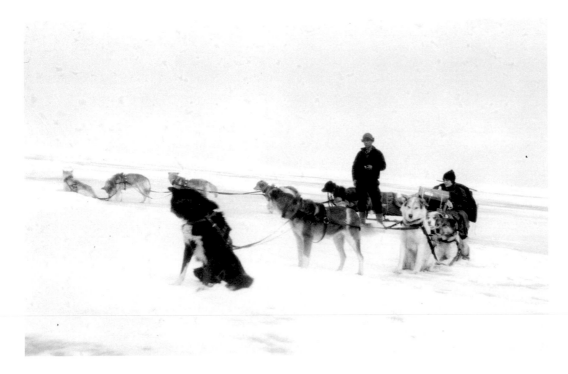

Left:
In winter, sleds drawn by husky dogs were sometimes the only mode of transport available in remote northern areas.

THE FIGHT FOR
PROFESSIONAL RECOGNITION

In the last two decades of the nineteenth century, nursing, by now a confident and effective profession, began to campaign for political and social recognition. On occasion, this led to fierce conflict, both within the profession and between its members and those of other groups. Many members of the profession were of a high social standing, and this meant that they were able to use their influence to effect change. Yet nursing, unlike medicine, also had many members from poorer social backgrounds, and the desire to accommodate the needs and recognize the roles of these less influential workers made the task of securing political recognition more complex.

The Work of Mrs Bedford Fenwick

The campaign for professionalization was led by the indomitable Mrs Bedford Fenwick. Born Ethel Gordon Manson in Elgin, Scotland, she received her nurse training at the Nottingham Children's Hospital and the Manchester Royal Infirmary. She then worked for eleven months as a ward sister at the London Hospital, before becoming Matron of St Bartholomew's Hospital in 1881, at the age of only twenty-four. Ethel was interested in developing nursing as a "scientific" discipline. She increased the length of training at St Bartholomew's from two to three years and developed a new system of instruction. In 1887 she married Dr Bedford Fenwick, a physician at the London Hospital. She then retired from nursing practice and began to campaign for nurse registration.

The desire among many nurses for a register of trained members of their profession was part of a drive to have their work recognized and their identity protected. A register would make sure that only those who had undertaken a recognized training would be given the title "nurse." This would not only raise the status of the profession, it would also protect the public from "amateurs." As nursing became more technical and scientific in focus, requiring a greater knowledge base and more expertise, it seemed to make sense to regulate its practice. Yet the push for registration raised issues and problems that had not been foreseen, and British elite nurses soon divided into two camps: one led by Mrs Bedford Fenwick, and the other by Eva Luckes, who had the influential support of Florence Nightingale. On Mrs Bedford Fenwick's side were powerful matrons such as Isla Stewart of St Bartholomew's and Catherine Wood of Great Ormond Street Children's Hospital, who wanted to see the technical and scientific side of nursing developed and recognized. On Luckes's side were those who feared that too great an emphasis on the scientific aspects of their work would turn nurses into mere technicians and would mean that the artistic side of their practice was lost.

Florence Nightingale did not get closely involved in the conflict but she did argue against a register by stating that it would turn nurses into mere "dictionaries." The challenge for the profession was to develop its knowledge and expertise and to obtain full professional recognition without losing its core identity as a compassionate art. These complexities meant that it would be more than twenty years before the battle for nurse registration was won.

The British Nurses' Association

The campaign for registration began in 1887 with the foundation of the British Nurses' Association. The Association, which was formally launched in 1888, quickly attracted a large membership and became very influential in the development of nursing practice. In 1891, it was allowed to call itself the Royal British Nurses' Association, and became the rallying point for all those who supported nurse registration. Ethel's fight was to be a long and sometimes bitter one: a register for nurses was not to be introduced until 1919.

Opposite:

*Mrs Bedford Fenwick
(1856–1947)
campaigned
for registration as
part of a drive among
nurses to realize their
power as practitioners
of a skilled profession.*

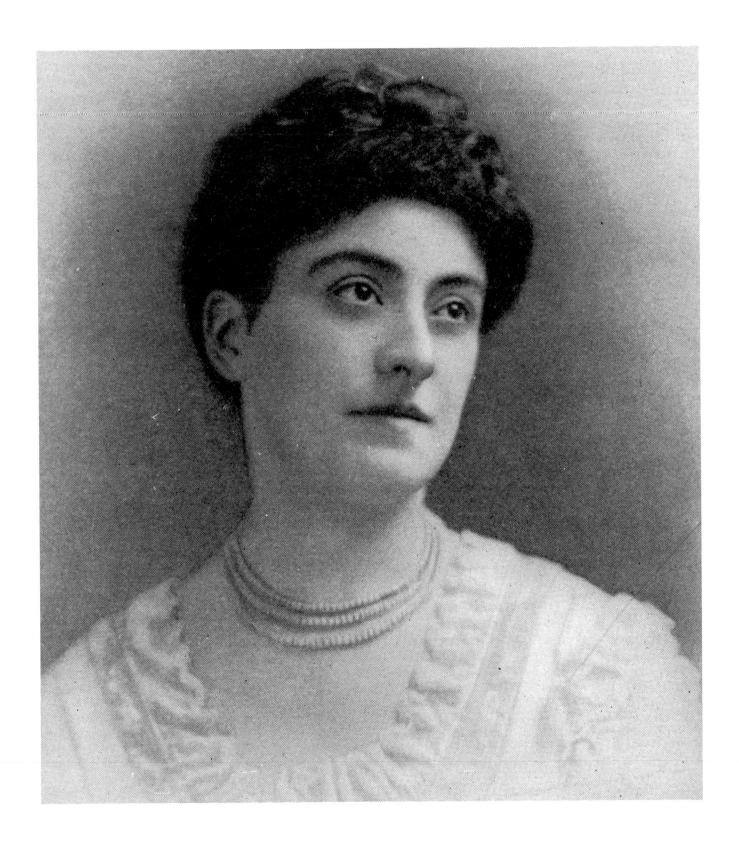

THE INTERNATIONAL COUNCIL OF NURSES

The International Council of Nurses was founded in 1899 with Mrs Bedford Fenwick as its president and Lavinia Dock as its honorary secretary. It modeled itself on the International Council of Women, with one association in each participating country. The Council became very influential in the development of nursing as a profession, permitting nurses of many countries to cooperate. For many years, its main office was in Oxford Street, London. In the twentieth century it moved its base to Geneva, Switzerland.

The great statement made by the foundation of the International Council of Nurses was that nursing, a nascent profession, had a common identity throughout the world. Its focus was on securing registration for nurses and maintaining high educational standards. By 1999 it had become a federation of 120 nursing associations from all parts of the globe, representing one and a half million nurses. In the year of its foundation, 1899, the Australasian Trained Nurses Association was also formed in Sydney, providing an additional focus for the development of nursing west of the Pacific Ocean.

Right:
Influential American nurse Lavinia Dock was the first Honorary Secretary of the International Council of Nurses.

Opposite:
In the late nineteenth century nurses in Australia were practicing independently in a range of clinical settings. The nurse here is based in the dispensary of an old hospital in Otway St Gundagai.

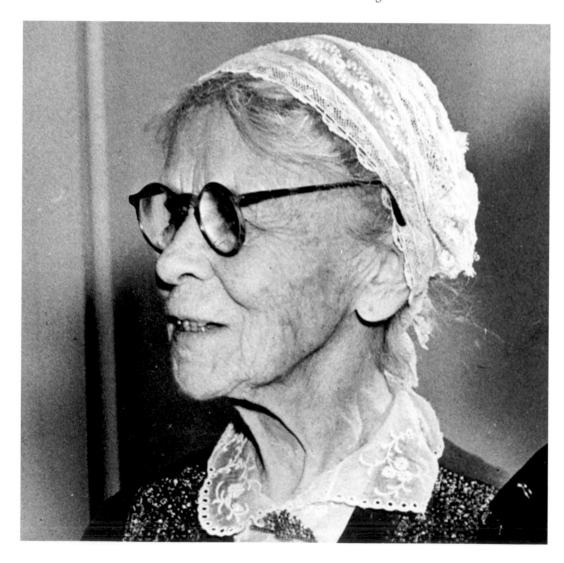

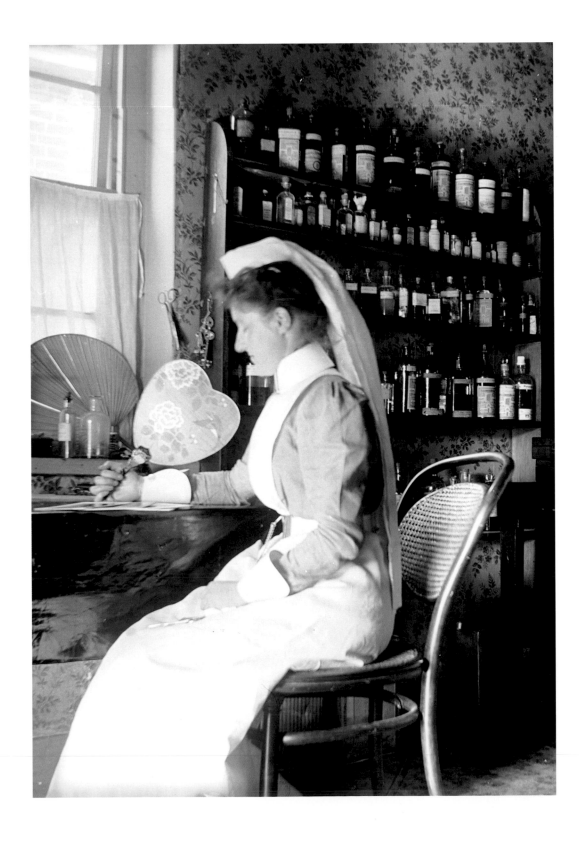

Testing Training

One of the ways in which nurses developed their practice during the nineteenth century was by creating formal training programs. From humble beginnings as a single series of lectures offered to the nurses in particular hospitals, these programs grew and developed into complex and detailed courses of theoretical and practical instruction of three years' duration. Although many hospitals and sisterhoods in Britain, the USA, Canada, and a number of other countries had ad hoc training programs in the early part of the nineteenth century, the Nightingale Training School, established in 1860, is often regarded as the first full formal secular (nonsectarian) school for nurses.

THE NIGHTINGALE TRAINING SCHOOL

The Nightingale Fund, which raised over £44,000 during 1856, the last year of the Crimean War, was controlled by Florence Nightingale and used to establish a training school for nurses. However, it was to take four years before the school opened at St Thomas's Hospital, London, England, in 1860. Florence believed that a nurse should be something very different from a doctor, and was therefore not sure how much involvement doctors should have in the training of nurses. She was also unsure about how much theory should be taught.

For Florence, nursing was as much about moral behavior as it was about technical knowledge and skill, so the selection of the right candidates was as important as their subsequent teaching and instruction. She believed that the nurses and the students (who were known as "probationers") in a hospital must be under the direct control of the Lady Superintendent, without interference from doctors or hospital governors, but it was difficult to find a hospital that would be suitable for such a project.

Eventually, the school was launched at St Thomas's Hospital under the direct control of Sarah Wardroper, the matron, with the resident medical

Right:
Isla Stewart, Matron of St Bartholomew's Hospital in England, wrote an important textbook for nurses. She believed that nurse training should develop along technical and scientific lines.

officer, Richard Whitfield, giving the lectures. In order to raise funds, wealthy probationers were given the title of "special probationer." This meant they were obliged to pay for their training, but in return could expect to be given positions as Sisters and Lady Superintendents when they qualified. Lower-class probationers did not pay. Florence wanted women without private wealth to be able to enter nursing, and some impoverished gentle-women were taken on as "specials," even if they were unable to pay.

In the early 1870s Florence introduced a "Home Sister," Elizabeth Torrance, and handed the medical teaching over to John Croft, a senior surgeon.

THE SPREAD OF THE NIGHTINGALE SYSTEM

Although the training at the Nightingale School was very unsystematic for decades after its foundation, Florence Nightingale's reputation ensured that it was highly regarded all over the world. Hospitals frequently asked for teams of nurses to be sent out from the school to develop nursing practice and education in their own institutions. In this way, the "Nightingale System of Nursing" was spread throughout the world.

At the same time, other influential London schools, such as those based at Guy's Hospital, St Bartholomew's Hospital, and the London Hospital, were developing their own training schools and their own views about how nursing practice should develop.

Below:
By the turn of the century, training schools had been developed in many hospitals throughout the UK. This photograph, showing a ward at King's College Hospital, demonstrates the importance of discipline and order in a hospital environment.

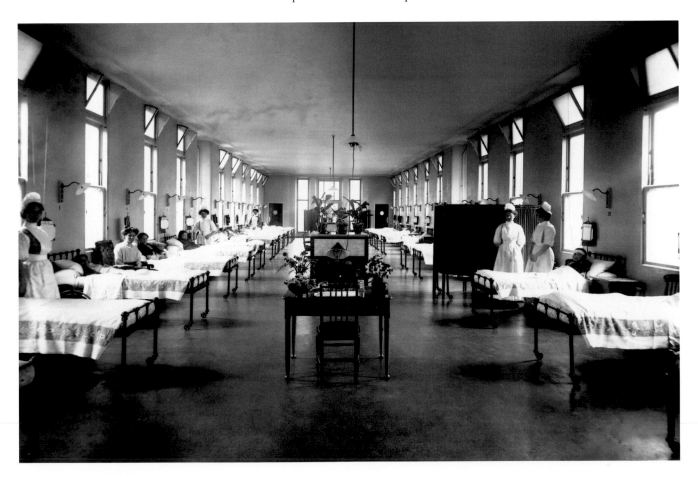

Angelique Pringle

One of Florence Nightingale's favorite trainees from St Thomas's—so much so, that Florence nicknamed her "The Pearl"—Angelique Pringle was appointed Deputy of the turbulent Edinburgh Royal Infirmary in 1872. The staff at the Infirmary were notoriously difficult to work with, and Angelique was sent there because of her expertise and diplomatic skill. In 1874 she became Superintendent of Nursing there in her own right. Following the retirement of Sarah Wardroper, Angelique was appointed Lady Superintendent of St Thomas's Hospital, where she remained until 1889, when she resigned in order to convert to Catholicism.

Rachel Williams

Another favored Nightingale probationer, Rachel Williams, was given the nickname "The Goddess." Rachel was said to have a sharp temper and a forthright tongue; she apparently did not have any qualms about getting into bitter disputes with doctors over the rights of Lady Superintendents to control the work and working conditions of nurses. She went to Edinburgh to support Angelique Pringle, but in 1876 was asked by Nightingale to apply for the position of Lady Superintendent of St Mary's Hospital, Paddington, London. In 1885 Rachel led a group of nurses to support the military expedition in Egypt and returned engaged to Mr Daniel Norris. She wrote a useful textbook for nurses, entitled *Norris's Nursing Notes*. She later became Superintendent of a nursing home in Cannes, France, and died there in 1908.

Lucy Osburn (1835–1891)

In 1866, Sir Henry Parkes, the then Colonial Secretary to New South Wales, wrote to Florence Nightingale, asking her to send a team of nurses to develop the Nightingale System in Sydney, Australia. Lucy Osburn was selected by Nightingale to lead a party of five nurses: Mary Barker, Eliza Blundell, Bessie Chant, Annie Miller, and Haldane Turriff. The choice was based largely on Lucy's high social standing—Lucy, in fact, had very little actual nurse training, but more than made up for this with her intrepid sense of adventure and love of travel. Some of her earliest nursing

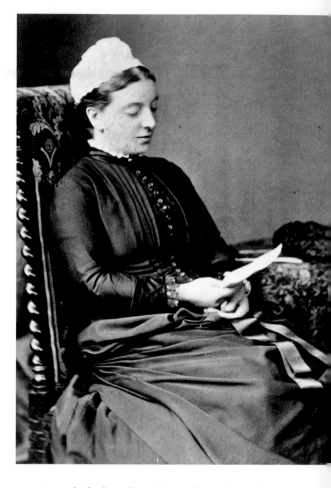

experience had taken place in Jerusalem, where she had also been known for her skill in taming horses.

Under the leadership of the previous matron, Bathsheba Ghost, the nursing at the Sydney Hospital had been unsystematic, but not entirely ineffective; some of the nurses there were, in Lucy's opinion, good. Although at first welcomed as a celebrity, Lucy later encountered some opposition. There was conflict with doctors and hospital governors, and Lucy was involved in a scandal involving Queen Victoria's second son, Prince Alfred, who had been wounded by an assassin and nursed back to health by the Nightingale nurses. Lucy's religious leanings also caused dismay, as many believed she was secretly a Catholic—in the 1860s and 1870s, the British fear of a Catholic revival was shared by Australian colonial society.

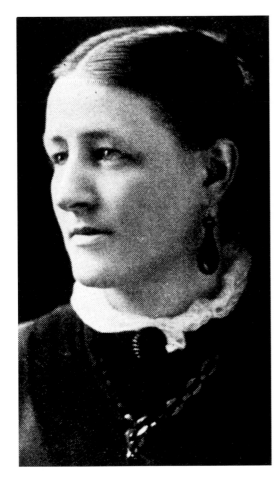

of typhoid during the first winter and others soon became ill. Maria came into conflict with the hospital authorities, who argued that she was spending too much money. After three years, the British nurses returned home.

Alice Fisher (1839–1888)

Born into a well-to-do family in Greenwich, England, in 1839, Alice Fisher was the well-educated daughter of an astronomer. Until her father's death in 1873, she lived a quiet life at home, writing novels and acting as his secretary. She then decided to enter nursing and became a paying lady probationer at the Nightingale School. Alice was one of the school's most successful and influential trainees. She went on to spread a particular vision of professional nursing. Fisher was Assistant Lady Superintendent of Nurses at Edinburgh Royal Infirmary from 1876–77. She was then Superintendent at the Newcastle Fever Hospital (1877), Addenbrooke's Hospital, Cambridge (1877–82), Radcliffe Infirmary, Oxford (1882), and Birmingham General Hospital (1882–84). In each hospital, she began a training school for nurses, funding these projects by laying off untrained nurses and hiring servants to do domestic work. This meant that nursing care was in the hands of trainees, who received no salary but were given their food and lodgings during the course of their training.

Alice was invited to take the role of Lady Superintendent to the Philadelphia General Hospital, USA, in 1884. She established a training school, and took on fifteen probationers. By opening up the nurses' lectures to the general public, Alice attracted further recruits and promoted her work to the public. Some of the lectures attracted huge audiences. Alice—a striking figure, almost 6 feet (1.8 meters) tall and with long red hair—was very popular in Philadelphia and did important work beyond the General Hospital. One of her most important projects was a campaign to reform the nursing care offered at the notorious "Old Blockley" Hospital. She died in 1888 of a heart attack, following a recurrence of rheumatic fever, first contracted at the Nightingale School.

Lucy remained as Matron of the Sydney Hospital until 1884, establishing and disseminating the Nightingale System of Nursing throughout New South Wales. She then returned to England, where she worked as a district nurse in Bloomsbury, London, caring for the sick poor. She was made Superintendent of the Southwark, Newington and Walworth District Nursing Association.

Maria Machin

In 1875 Florence Nightingale sent a team of five nurses to Montreal, Canada, at the request of the administrators of the city's general hospital. They were led by Maria Machin—a Canadian by birth who had trained at the Nightingale School. The intention had been to establish a training school there. Unfortunately, however, the conditions at the hospital were so poor that one of the team died

THE AMERICAN SCHOOLS

The development of the great nurse training schools in the USA gained pace rapidly from the 1870s onward. Among the most important and influential were the schools at the Philadelphia General Hospital; the Massachusetts General Hospital, Boston; the Bellevue Hospital, New York; the Connecticut Training School, New Haven; and the Johns Hopkins Hospital, Baltimore.

The nurse–doctor relationship has had a rather tortuous history in America, as in Britain, and the attitude of the medical profession had an important influence on the development of nurse training. Some doctors frankly opposed the organization and training of nursing, seeing nurses as interfering with their medical work. Others saw nurses as useful and recognized the good they did in assisting patients' recovery. Yet even those with a more positive view saw nursing as subordinate to medicine, and tended to view nurses as their own "handmaidens."

At Bellevue and other hospitals, the establishment of nursing was opposed by doctors, until they realized that nursing not only helped patients, but assisted and promoted their own work too. By contrast, in some hospitals, such as the New Haven Hospital, Connecticut, it was doctors themselves who, from the start, established and promoted the nurse training school. The New Haven school was, however, unusual since it was established outside the hospital as a separate organization, but offered students the opportunity to gain practice on the wards. One of its achievements was the publication of its own, highly influential textbook of nursing, written jointly by nurses and doctors.

The Boston training school at the Massachusetts General Hospital was able to build on a tradition of good nursing by working-class women. The Women's Educational Union worked to develop the training school there, drawing on the support of influential physicians Gill Wylie and Susan Dimock. The proposals met with opposition, and were only introduced, initially, on an experimental basis in 1873. In 1874, Linda Richards was appointed Superintendent of Nurses. She developed a lecture program and a system of training, eventually winning over medical opinion and having the school recognized as an integral part of the hospital.

Nurse Training at Bellevue

The establishment of a training school for nurses at the Bellevue Hospital, New York, was one of the most difficult nursing reforms ever achieved. In 1871 a women's visiting committee recommended the establishment of some form of nurse training at the hospital, but the proposal was opposed by Bellevue's Medical Board and nothing was done. In 1872 the philanthropist and welfare worker Louisa Lee Schuyler founded the New York State Charities Aid Association, with visiting committees empowered to inspect the local hospitals. When one such committee visited Bellevue, the truth about conditions there was discovered.

It was found that, in the main, nursing care was carried out by ex-convicts with no training. Many did their best to offer comfort to patients, but others bullied and embezzled money from those in their care. There were no night nurses, merely a night watchman, and even during the day, each nurse had to care for up to thirty patients. Infectious diseases and wound-sepsis were rife and many patients died needlessly. Although the hospital's Board of Governors still opposed calls for reform, one of the hospital's interns, Dr Gill Wylie, offered to go to Europe and seek advice from Florence Nightingale, among others. His report on European training schools was to prove influential in the establishment of a number of American schools.

Eventually, Miss Schuyler managed to establish an experimental training course for nurses in six of the wards at Bellevue. Charitable funds were used to establish a nursing home, and the training school at Bellevue made its first, shaky beginnings. A Miss Bowden, known as Sister Helen, who was a member of the All Saints' Sisterhood in Baltimore, and who had trained at University College Hospital, London, was appointed Superintendent. Sister Helen was a remarkable woman whose force of character allowed her to develop the practice of nursing at Bellevue. She did so in the face of political opposition and the fatalistic disapproval of doctors, who thought that no well-educated woman would be able to cope with the difficulties of caring for patients from the squalid backstreets of New York. At first, their pessimism seemed well founded. Of the first seventy-three applicants, only twenty-nine were thought suitable for training and only six successfully completed the one-year course and one year's probation. Yet even

though the odds seemed to be stacked against its success, the nurse training school gained a foothold, and these first six nurses graduated in May 1875. In 1874 Linda Richards (see page 65) became the hospital's Night Superintendent, and began the practice of record-keeping among the nurses. Eventually, the doctors were won around, as they realized that the competence of the nurses would make more complex medical and surgical procedures possible. The nurses found that their work was now admired and respected.

Below:
Despite its inauspicious beginnings, by the late nineteenth century the Bellevue Hospital training school was one of the most highly respected in the USA.

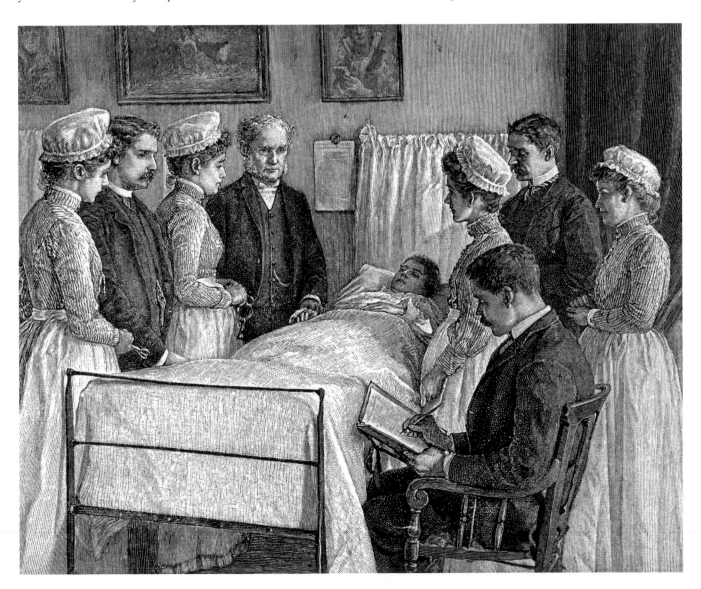

TRAINING SCHOOLS IN EUROPE

The mid-nineteenth century saw the emergence of secular training schools throughout Europe.

France

In the 1870s there were calls for the development of secular nursing schools to replace the monopoly hitherto held by regular and secular religious orders. The earliest such schools were developed successfully in Paris in 1878. In 1899, following increasing support for secular training from the French government, some hospitals expelled all their nursing nuns, while others strove to retain the expertise of their religious sisters, incorporating it into the development of new schools.

Germany and Scandinavia

Many famous nurses had visited Germany's best-known nursing institution, the Kaiserswerth (see page 37). As the century advanced, however, religious sisterhoods began to lose their influence and secular training schools were opened in Berlin and Hamburg in the 1880s and 1890s. In 1903 the German Nurses' Association was founded by Agnes Karll.

In Scandinavia the Deaconess Institution, run along Kaiserswerth lines, was founded in Stockholm in 1851, and in 1884, a small home for nurses grew into the "Sophia Home," a large training school where nurses could live and train on one site. Nursing developed along similar lines in Denmark, Norway, and Finland, with deaconess movements protecting the discipline of nursing and new training institutions developing it further. The Danish Nurses Organization, founded in 1899, was one of the earliest nurses' associations in the world.

Italy and Spain

In Italy and Spain, religious influences were strong throughout the nineteenth century. In Spain, the first secular training school was established at the Instituto Rubio, Madrid. Conditions were strict and the organization resembled a religious order, until Marie Zomal took over in 1910 and introduced new reforms. In Italy, hospitals were run by religious orders until the end of the century, when the influence of a small number of reformers began to be felt. Among them was the British nurse Grace Baxter, who established the Blue Cross Nursing School in Naples in 1900.

Right:
A group of Spanish nurses from the first secular nurse training school established in Madrid, Spain. Third from the right is Marie Zomal, who took over the directorship of the school in 1910. An experienced nurse who had trained in Berlin, Marie greatly improved nursing conditions with her reforms, which included reducing work hours and modernizing uniforms.

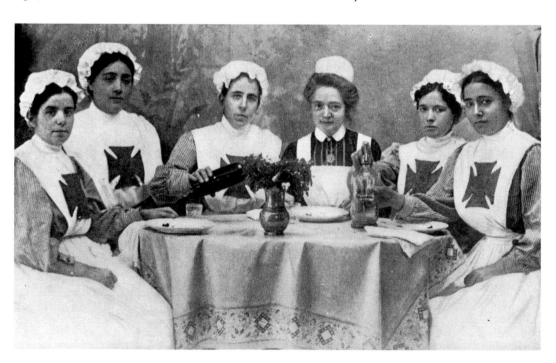

THE TRANSMISSION OF KNOWLEDGE

As the knowledge that a woman required to be an effective nurse expanded, the need to draw it together into textbooks and training manuals became very clear. Two of the most important textbooks to emerge from Great Britain at the end of the century were *General Nursing*, written by Eva Luckes, Matron of the London Hospital, and *Practical Nursing*, by Isla Stewart, Matron of St Bartholomew's Hospital, London.

The purpose of these books was not only to instruct nurses, but also to promote both the expertise and the moral qualities of the nurse and make her work more widely understood. Their writers made great claims for the special qualities of nurses in an era when it was believed that some women were "born nurses." In *Practical Nursing*, Isla Stewart argued that:

"To become a good nurse, a woman must possess considerable intelligence, a good education, healthy physique, good manners, an even temper, a sympathetic temperament, and deft clever hands. To these she must add habits of observation, punctuality, obedience, cleanliness, a sense of

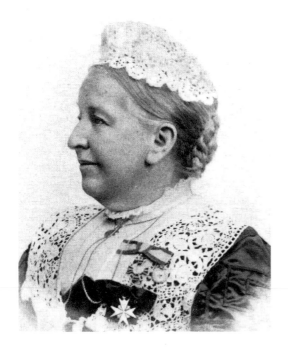

proportion, and a capacity for and habit of accurate statement. Training can only strengthen these qualities and habits; it cannot produce them."

Toward the end of the nineteenth century, nursing became more and more complex and technical, and there was a risk that the work of nurses would be split into two halves. On the one hand, there was the caring work, which had been passed on since time immemorial from teacher to apprentice. On the other, there were the new technical skills and knowledge, deriving from nineteenth-century science, which were becoming an increasing part of the nurse's work. In their textbooks, leaders of the profession debated the changes that were taking place rapidly in nursing practice. Eva Luckes was one of those who argued passionately that nursing must not lose sight of its identity as a caring art. In the Preface to the second edition of her book, *General Nursing*, she wrote of her concern that the technical side of nursing was being overrated:

"The inevitable result of this is to concentrate attention chiefly on the mechanical side of Nursing and to regard the human side of the work as a secondary consideration. Those who aim to become Nurses merely by book knowledge and examinations can, at best, only become machines. Their presence will bring no sense of comfort to those who are suffering, or to those who are anxiously watching every turn of their illness."

These issues were further debated in the earliest professional journals. In Britain, the *Nursing Record* (later renamed the *British Journal of Nursing*) was the first to emerge, followed by the *Nursing Times* and *Nursing Mirror*. In the USA, the *American Journal of Nursing* rapidly became influential, while in Australia, the *Australasian Nurses' Journal* gave widely scattered communities of nurses a sense of identity. Many of these early journals have enjoyed uninterrupted circulation until the present day. Nursing was clearly asserting itself as a developing profession.

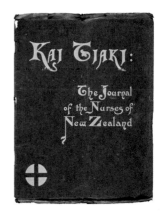

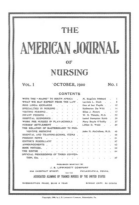

Above:

Top *Cover of an early issue of the New Zealand journal,* Kai Tiaki.

Bottom *Cover of the first issue of* The American Journal of Nursing.

Left:

Eva Luckes was the indomitable Matron of the London Hospital for more than two decades. Her textbook, General Nursing, *had an important influence on the development of nurse-training throughout the world.*

The Emergence of Surgical Nursing

The greatest scientific discovery of the nineteenth century was germ theory. In the last three decades of the century, Robert Koch in Germany and Louis Pasteur in France identified the microscopic creatures—invisible to the naked eye—that caused healthy processes such as the fermentation of wine, and unhealthy ones such as disease. As infection became an accepted aspect of human life, infection control emerged as an important nursing role. At the same time the discovery of anesthesia permitted more and more complex surgery to be performed, and surgical nursing emerged as a specialism. Using "Listerian antisepsis," and later asepsis, to prevent wound infection, as well as learning meticulous routines to monitor patient safety, nurses were essential to patient survival.

HYGIENE, ANTISEPSIS, AND ASEPSIS

The discovery of the germ meant that nurses developed their practice in ways that could control and destroy infectious diseases. Nurses had been interested in cleanliness and hygiene for decades, but their actions had been driven by a belief in the existence of "miasmas"—tiny particles of foul and dangerous airborne matter. Until 1885, Florence Nightingale was a strong believer in the "miasma theory," and this influenced nurses to see the causes of disease in a similar way. Consequently, trained nurses were already taking the lead in ward hygiene by the time the German physician Robert Koch discovered the anthrax and tubercle bacilli in the 1880s. They already believed that a scrupulously clean and well-aired ward would always be a healthy ward. Nurses had direct supervision of ward maids and accepted ultimate responsibility for the cleanliness of the environment.

Cleanliness and order were part of the image of purity that was projected by the nurse herself. It sent patients the message that they would be safe in her care; starched collars and cuffs, white aprons, and neat caps symbolized the nurse as the guardian of her patient's health. Nurses, both in hospital and in the community, were seen as "sanitary missioners" who were on a crusade to ensure health through cleanliness and morality. As germ theory gained ground, measures that had been used to control miasma now became important in destroying germs. It became clear that germs thrived in dirty environments, and it was not difficult for nurses to see that they were no longer controlling the environment in order to prevent miasmas; they were now controlling it in order to eradicate germs. Although in theory this meant a great conceptual leap, in reality it meant very little change to their sanitary practices.

But hygiene was not the only aspect of the nurse's role that kept patients safe. In a world now known to be full of germs, surgeons radically changed their ways of working in order to avoid giving their patients infectious diseases during surgery. They did so in ways that would not have been possible had nurses not been there to help them. Two practices emerged at the end of the nineteenth century: antisepsis—the use of chemicals with germ-killing properties; and asepsis—a range of measures designed to keep the environment completely clear of germs. Nurses were pivotal in ensuring these practices were followed safely.

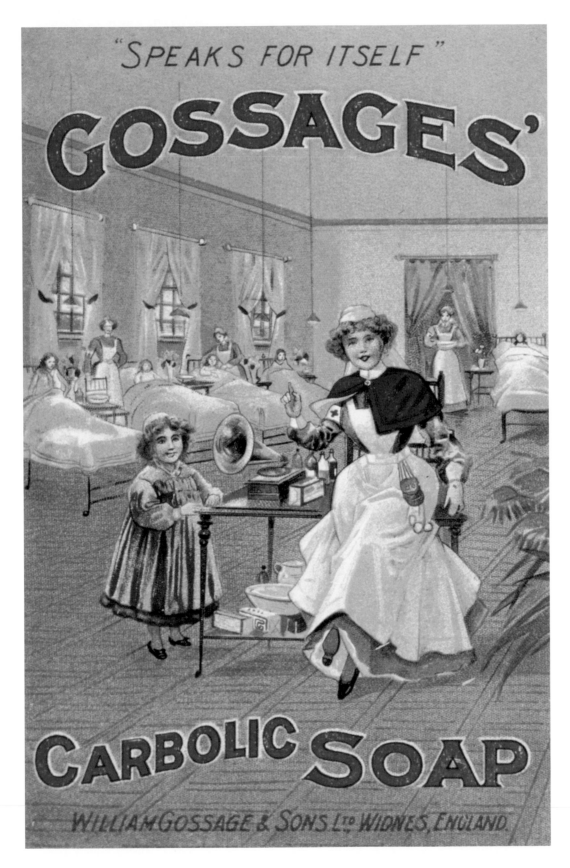

Left:
At the turn of the century strong emphasis was placed on ward hygiene. This advertisement for carbolic soap draws on the image of the nurse to make its appeal.

Nursing textbooks written after the mid 1880s began to include information on how to prevent infection, and many offered explanations of germ theory and antisepsis. Rachel Norris (previously Rachel Williams) had been Acting Superintendent of the Royal Military Hospital at Suez, and had also worked as Matron of St Mary's Hospital, London. In her book, *Norris's Nursing Notes*, she explained that:

"Antiseptic Surgery is based upon the theory that putrefaction is due to the presence of microscopic germs in the air, in water, on the clothes, or on the hands, in fact, upon everything that is not in itself antiseptic. It is thought that putrefaction is, perhaps, the greatest cause of mischief in open wounds."

The man who is given the credit for being the first to discover antisepsis is Joseph Lister, a Quaker born in London in 1827, who gained his medical education at University College, London. While practicing at the Edinburgh Royal Infirmary, Lister experimented with the use of carbolic acid to kill germs during surgery. In 1865 he perfected the technique of using an apparatus that would spray carbolic over the surface of a wound while the surgeon was operating, thus killing germs as they entered the field of operation. The technique was a complex one that required skilled assistance from "theater nurses."

After surgery, nurses often cared for patients' wounds (though surgeon's assistants known as "dressers" could also be involved in this work). Carbolic acid was often used during dressing-changes, just as it was for operations. Many complex dressings were changed every day.

Eventually, asepsis—the complete elimination of germs from a surgical procedure—became the norm, and antisepsis was used only as a safety net, to kill any germs that entered by accident. At the end of the century, Isla Stewart, Matron of St Bartholomew's Hospital, emphasized the importance of asepsis in her book, *Practical Nursing*.

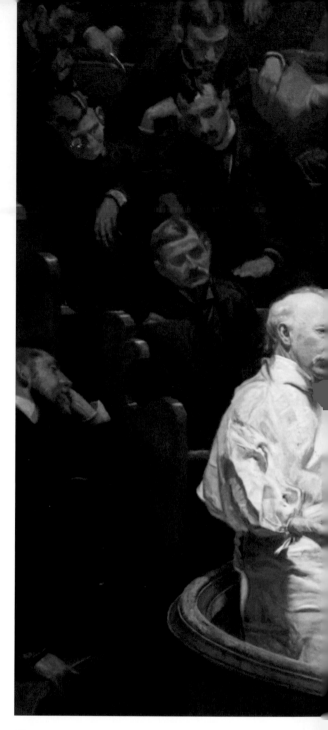

Above:
The Agnew Clinic
(1889) by Thomas Eakins.
Famous American surgeon
Dr D. Hayes Agnew is
depicted performing a
mastectomy, assisted
by medical staff and
Nurse Mary U. Clymer.

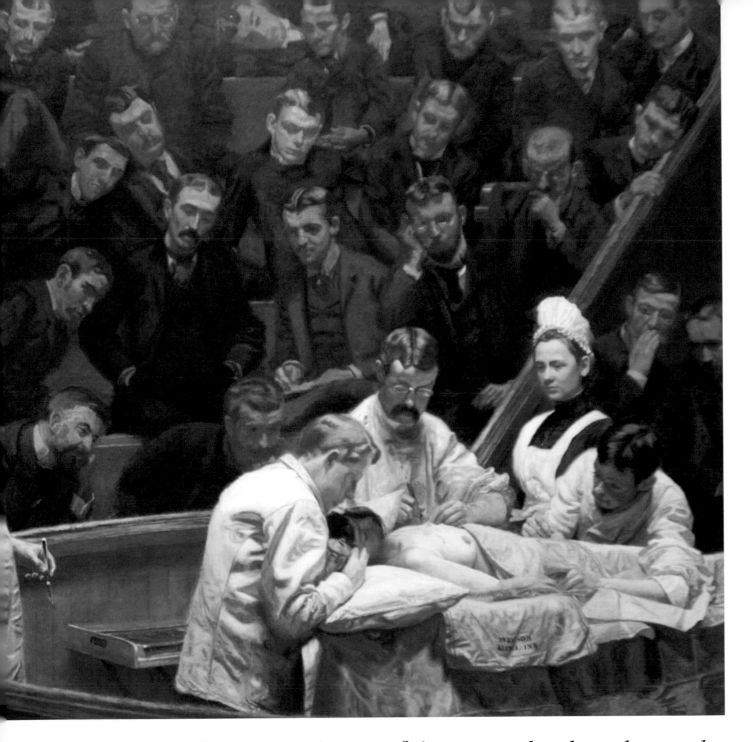

"The success of the surgical nurse of the present day depends entirely on her ability to understand and appreciate the theory of 'asepsis,' or surgical cleanliness, which underlies the practice of modern surgery, and her capacity for intelligent attention to the minutest details."

Isla Stewart

Practical Nursing (1899–1903)

ANESTHESIA

Of equal importance to the discovery of asepsis and antisepsis was the invention of the general anesthetic in the 1040s. Anesthesia meant that surgery could be done without the excruciating pain that went with the tortuous processes of cutting into a patient's body. It also meant that surgery was much more likely to be successful, because a patient was much less likely to die of shock, and also the surgeon could take his time and conduct the operation with care. The first anesthetic was ether. Later, chloroform was used. Both substances caused extreme vomiting and were also likely to place the patient at some risk of pneumonia. This meant a great deal of work for nurses, who prepared patients for surgery and cared for them after their return from the operating theater.

Nurses made sure that patients who were to undergo surgery took no food or drink for at least six hours. This would prevent vomiting and reduce the danger that the patient might choke when emerging from the effects of anesthesia. When patients returned to their wards following surgery, nurses made them comfortable, cared for them through the devastating temporary illness and disorientation that anesthesia caused, and monitored them closely. The pulse, blood pressure, and temperature were taken at regular intervals and wounds were checked for bleeding or suppuration. By their close care and attention, nurses made sure that patients did not die from surgical procedures, and surgeons knew that, without efficient, effective nurses, it would be impossible for them to conduct most of the complex procedures that gave them their heroic status in the late nineteenth century.

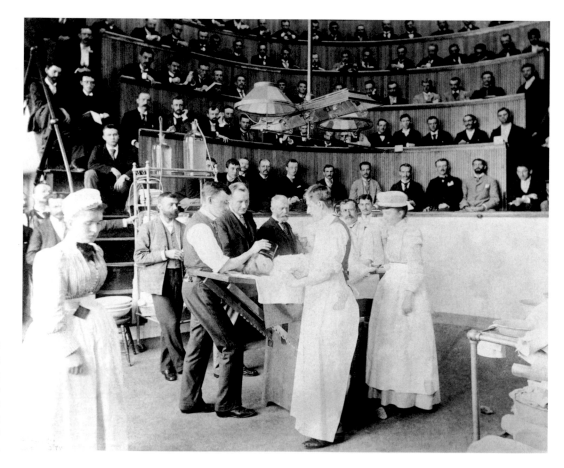

Right:
Operating theaters were important teaching scenarios in the nineteenth century. Here three nurses are shown assisting at an operation in Manhattan in 1898.

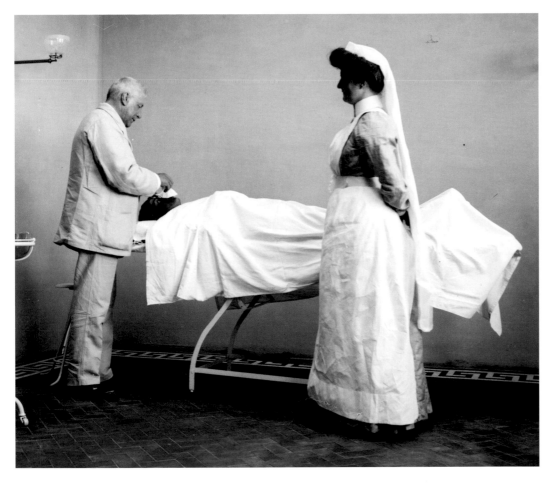

*In this photograph taken
in an Australian hospital
at the turn of the century,
a nurse looks on while an
anesthetist attends
to a patient.*

THE LYNCHPIN OF SURGICAL PRACTICE

By the end of the nineteenth century nursing practice was being rapidly transformed. Nurses were an integral part of the revolutionary changes that had been taking place throughout the century, in a process that became known as the "birth of the clinic." The French philosopher Michel Foucault has identified this process as one in which the medical expert became all-powerful and the patient became a mere "object" on whom he practiced his science. What has not often been recognized is the role of the nurse in these processes. The expert and skilled day-to-day work of nurses won no awards and has found its way into very few congratulatory histories. Yet it was nurses who were supporting and protecting both patients and surgeons as they navigated the dangerous territories of medical innovation. Sometimes nurses protested against the treatment of patients as experimental objects. In the Paris Hôtel Dieu, for example, Daughters of Charity spoke out against the tendency of surgeons to "try out" new procedures on poor and powerless patients. For the most part, though, by the turn of the century, nurses and doctors were practicing harmoniously together for the good of their patients.

The nineteenth century had been a century of dramatic change for nursing. Those who nursed the sick had been transformed during its course from a downtrodden, poorly paid, and reviled group of outcasts, to a highly respected profession whose members had a clear sense of their own place in society. The scene was set for the further development of their profession in the turbulent twentieth century.

Caps

Nurses' caps reflect the changing story of nursing. They show how nurses were perceived, and what their role in society was at different times. The earliest nurses' headdresses evolved from the nun's coif; early versions were often made from starched, white material. In some of the late-nineteenth-century hospitals, particularly in the USA, nurses wore a mob or maid's style cap that was influenced by the caps worn by domestic servants. Today nurses wear hygienic, often brightly colored and printed scrub caps. The change to scrubs in the late twentieth century was, in part, an attempt to maintain hygiene and cleanliness, but it was also part of the drive to attract more men into the profession.

As nursing started to develop as a discipline in the nineteenth century, nurses began to establish their identity as a secular profession. Caps became sharper and less flowing than the previous coifs. Although they still held symbolic value, caps were now an essentially practical part of the nurse's uniform. Usually made from cotton or linen, they were carefully starched and neatly folded. As germ theory emerged, the purpose of the cap was, increasingly, to hold the hair away from the face and shoulders, to allow a clearer field of view when intricate work was being undertaken, and to prevent contamination of sterile work-fields. And yet, caps did also retain a symbolic status. Military nurses in many countries retained a nun-like veil to denote their purity and set them apart from the chaos of war. This was essentially protective. In many parts of the world, but especially in the USA, "capping ceremonies" formed the rites of passage through which individuals graduated from student to staff nurse. Unique and sometimes very intricate styles of cap were designed by individual hospitals to give their own nurses a clear identity, and colors or stripes were used to indicate grade, status, or seniority.

Nurses' caps are an intriguing element of their uniform. Carrying multiple meanings—from cleanliness and hygiene, through efficiency and purity, to femininity—the cap has always set nurses apart from other professions. Although similar "scrub caps" are worn today by all health professionals, color and style are still often used to establish the separate identity of nurses.

From left to right:

The development of the nurse's cap, from nun's veil to mob cap.

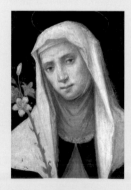 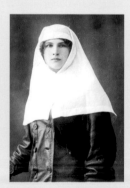 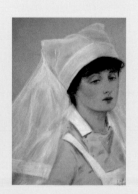 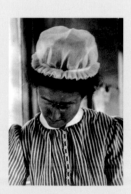

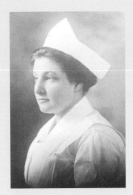

Above:
An early starched cap.

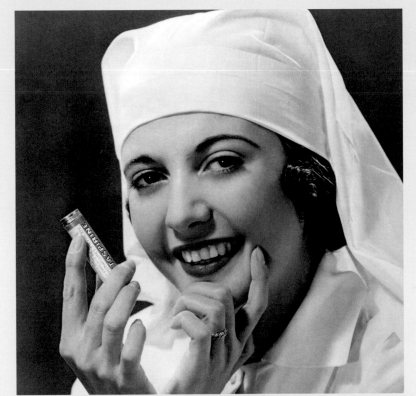

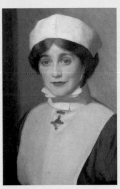

Above:
Portrait of a nurse belonging to the St John's Ambulance Association, 1917.

Left:
A 1950s French advertisement for aspirin. The veil did not disappear completely until the latter half of the twentieth century.

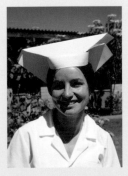

Above:
A mortar board influenced design worn by a Hamersley Iron company nurse in Western Australia, 1974.

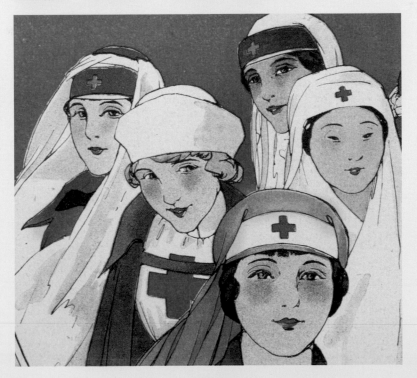

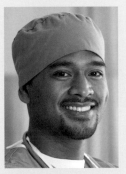

Above:
A 21st-century scrub cap.

Left:
Illustration from the French magazine La Baïonnette, October 1915, bearing the legend "The prettiest fashion because nurses of all countries have adopted it."

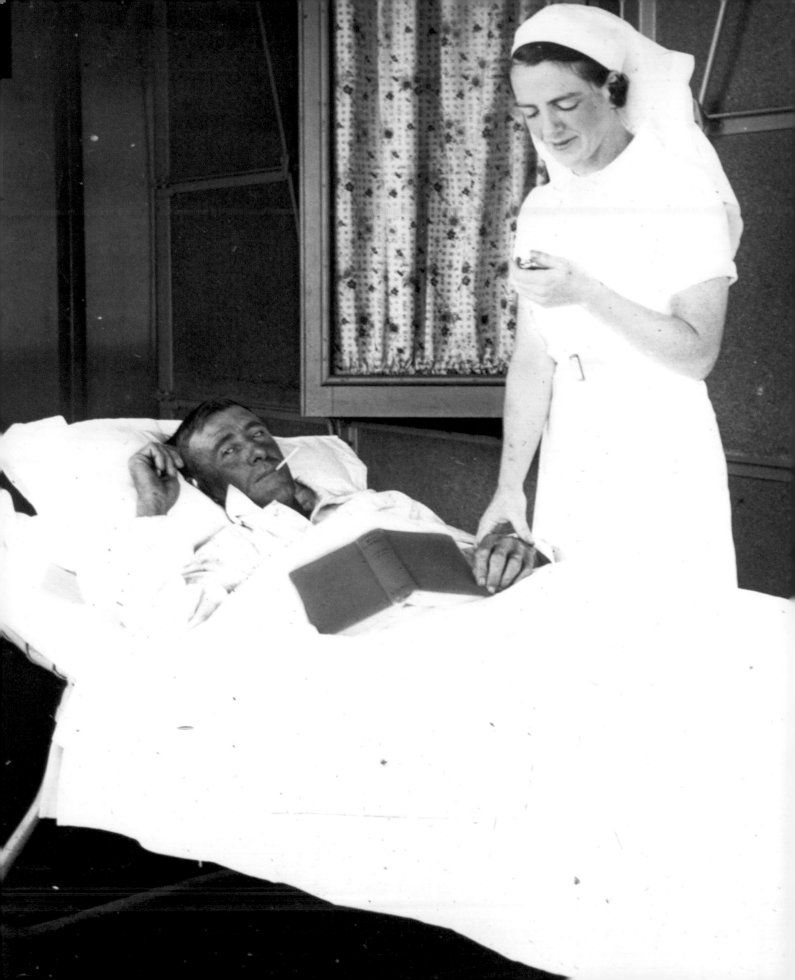

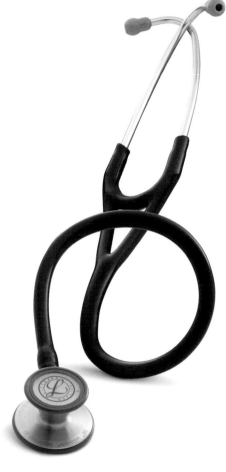

THE TWENTIETH CENTURY

3

Official recognition and new nursing theories were to bring greater autonomy and an increasing role in the fight against disease. Groundbreaking medical advances eradicated some illnesses completely, but for each battle that was fought and won, a new challenge emerged, as nursing fought to keep pace with an ever-changing world.

The March of Change

Although the nineteenth century had seen great changes in the nursing profession throughout the world, as the new century opened nurses were still fighting for official recognition. In Britain, the registration debate that had begun in the 1880s was still continuing amid great opposition. In 1916, the College of Nursing was formed to give nurses a forum for debate on the development of their discipline. The college later gained a royal charter. It became a trade union for nurses, protecting them as they navigated the dangerous twentieth-century territories of practice-settings that combined chronic staff shortages with impressive but often risky medical innovations. Nevertheless, for most countries there was to be a long wait before the nursing profession gained formal recognition.

NURSE REGISTRATION

Registration to distinguish trained nurses from untrained nursing assistants was fundamental in the fight for nurses' official recognition. It is widely believed that New Zealand was the first country to pass legislation to register nurses in 1901. However, it should be noted that South African nurses were registered under the Cape Medical Council from 1891.

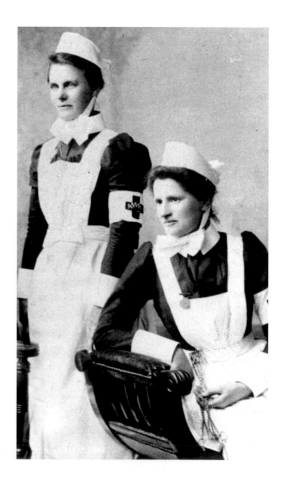

The earliest American state to gain registration was North Carolina (1903). By 1910, twenty states had passed legislation to register nurses. The protracted struggle for registration in Britain was finally won with the passing of the Nurses' Registration Act in December 1919. Queensland, Australia, introduced a register in 1912 and other Australian provinces followed over the next ten years, as did approximately thirty other countries. Norway was one of the last states to introduce legislation, not obtaining its own register until 1949. By this date, most countries also had a Division or Section for nursing within their Health Ministries.

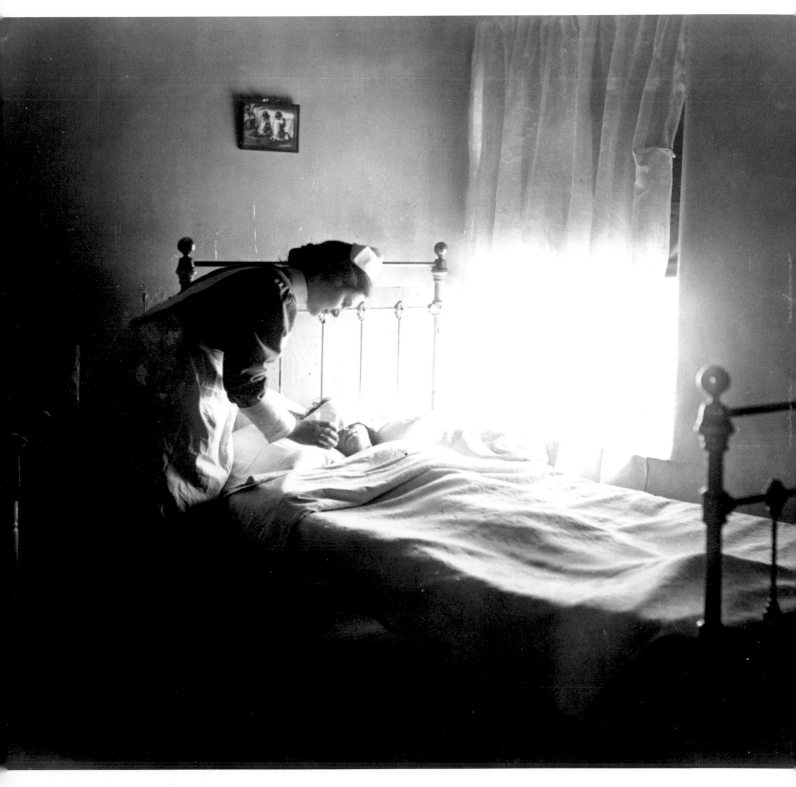

NURSING IN A CHANGING WORLD

During the course of the twentieth century dramatic changes took place in the health of the world's populations, and nurses in the developed world saw their workload change rapidly. Until the late 1940s, large numbers of their patients had suffered from life-threatening infectious diseases. Following the introduction of antibiotics, death rates from these conditions fell, and there was a sense of optimism—a belief that medical science might eventually be able to eradicate disease entirely. But sadly such optimism proved unfounded. New waves of chronic diseases emerged, partly because people lived long enough to contract them, but also because the inherently unhealthy lifestyles of affluent societies gave rise to chronic ill health. In the second half of the century, as death rates from infection fell, mortality and morbidity rates for cancers, heart disease, vascular disease, and respiratory conditions rose dramatically.

The emergence of these diseases led to major changes in the way nurses worked. Nurses in hospitals now did less of the labor-intensive work associated with caring for patients with acute fevers, such as bathing and sponging, giving food and fluids, and offering comfort and relief during periods of delirium or exhaustion. Instead, they were confronted with a highly unstable hospital population, none of whose members were going through the "crisis" of fever, but any of whom could "collapse" at any moment. Patients with heart disease, in particular, could suffer a myocardial infarction (heart attack) with no warning, and those with respiratory conditions might go into respiratory arrest and stop breathing. In such cases, nurses had to be capable of making very rapid judgments and acting quickly.

The twentieth-century nurse had to have a deep understanding of the physiological processes taking place inside patients' bodies, and the capacity to begin emergency treatment whether a doctor was present or not. They also had to understand the complexities of their patients' treatments—both medical and surgical.

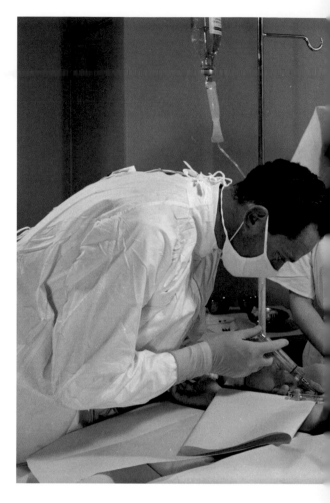

THE INDEPENDENCE
OF NURSING PRACTICE

Nurses were beginning to act much more independently. Although much of their practice depended on "doctors' orders," they were now working jointly with doctors to decide their patients' treatments, and were competent to modify these within an agreed range.

In addition to dealing with patients with unstable heart and respiratory function, nurses were also working in hospitals where very complex surgery was carried out to combat the malignant diseases that seemed so often to be associated with affluent lifestyles. Cancers, if they had not spread, could be excised—literally cut from the body by a surgeon. But these processes were highly dangerous, and

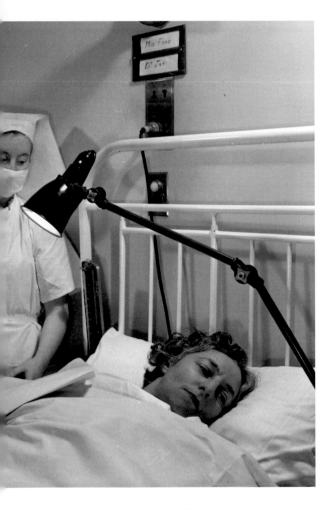

> "*The nursing practice
> and education reforms of
> the 1960s and 1970s
> broke with the status
> quo, ignored laws
> governing nursing, and
> insisted that patients had
> a right to all that nurses
> had to offer.*"

Joan Lynaugh

Professor Emerita, University of Pennsylvania

patients had to be closely monitored by nurses, both before and after surgery. Patients emerging from anesthesia after an operation were in a fragile state—their condition could deteriorate rapidly at any time. Nurses monitored their pulse, blood pressure, and temperature, and cared for them until the effects of the anesthetic had worn off. They also ensured that the patient's pain was under control at all times—no easy task following traumatic surgery.

When patients with chronic diseases could not be cured—as was very often the case—nurses were there to help and support them through the long and painful process of death. No longer a dramatic episode lasting just a few days while waiting for the crisis of fever to break or for the patient to die,

disease was now a long-drawn-out process. Death from cancer was painful and slow, taking place over several months. Nurses became expert in understanding the needs of dying patients: their knowledge of pain relief, emotional support, and spiritual care for these patients increased dramatically, as they developed their specialist knowledge of "palliative care."

And finally there were those individuals who lived into old age without suffering from any really acute episodes of disease, but who became frail and dependent. Care of the elderly became an increasingly important specialism during the twentieth century. Unfortunately, because it was not associated with "high-tech" innovation, or life-saving techniques, and because no dramatic stories could be told about its wonders, it was—and continues to be—a desperately underfunded area of care. In wards for the elderly, the greatest work of the nurse involved using her own ingenuity to provide good, supportive care with very few resources.

VISITING NURSES IN THE USA

In the 1950s, hospitals were becoming larger and the care offered in them more technical. Yet there was an increasing realization that a patient's own home was the safest place for recovery from illness—a policy that was also seen as "cost effective" in an era of soaring health-care costs. After the introduction of Medicare in 1965, visiting nursing services expanded dramatically throughout the USA. During the second half of the century, patients would be discharged increasingly early from hospital after treatment or surgery. This brought challenges for home-care nurses, who now had to handle high-tech equipment and carry out life-threatening treatments in the uncontrolled environment of a patient's home.

Visiting nurses gave injections and other medications, performed complex dressings, and undertook a range of technical procedures, from putting in eyedrops to giving blood transfusions. But they were not merely technicians. They also gave core nursing care to the seriously ill, keeping them comfortable and clean, and preventing pressure sores, as well as offering instruction on particular conditions and treatments and general advice on keeping well.

Public Health Nursing

As the twentieth century began, public health nursing was becoming more organized and specialized in many developed countries. In the USA, Visiting Nurse Associations developed, and superintendents were employed to run the services they offered. "Neighborhood nursing" allowed each nurse to work as a general practitioner in a distinct neighborhood. Such nurses generally worked a six-day week, from Monday to Saturday. A typical day was eight to ten hours long, and nurses visited patients ranging from the very sick, who they saw twice a day, to those with chronic complaints such as bronchitis, who needed care and medication, and those with wounds and ulcers that needed to be dressed. Nurses took their equipment and medicines everywhere with them in a black bag, and, later in the century, also carried more complex equipment such as portable sterilizers and oxygen cylinders.

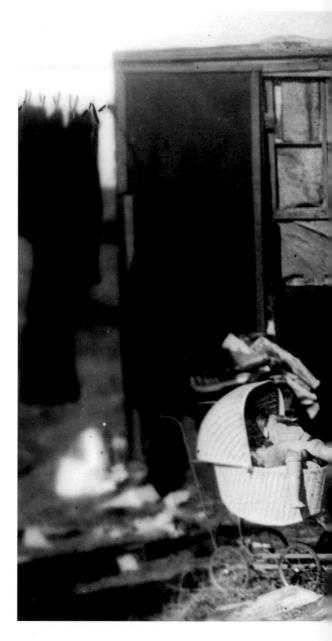

In the ever-increasing battle to eradicate diseases of affluence, public health nurses educated people about the dangers of unhealthy habits such as smoking, overeating, and excessive drinking. Health education in the second half of the twentieth century was, in many ways, more difficult than it had been in the first half—the messages had to be subtler, and the focus had to be on empowering people to

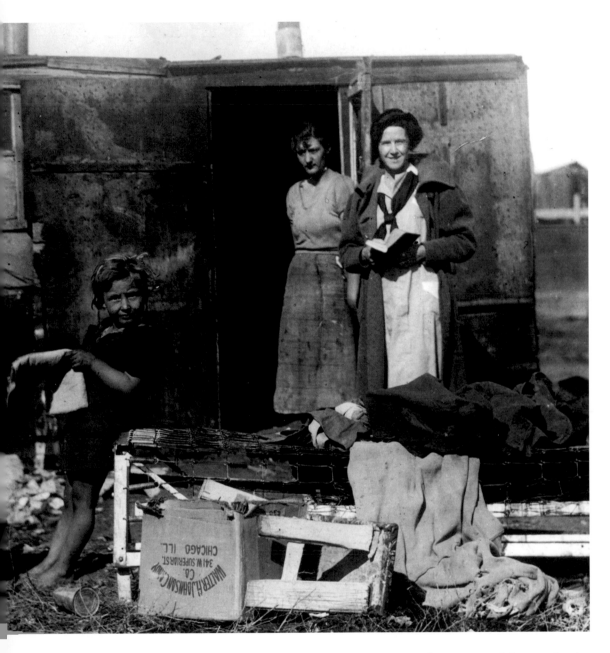

In rural areas, public health nurses were viewed as "mothers' friends."
They were allies in the battle against hardship and deprivation, bringing public health knowledge and practical nursing care to impoverished households.

change their behavior, rather than on simply giving them information.

Yet even as diseases of affluence were taking hold, many people still lived in conditions of abject poverty. Nurses continued to support these poorer members of society, helping them to understand the risks associated with poor hygiene or inade-

quate nutrition. They recognized that simply educating an impoverished family, without giving it the means to support itself, was not enough; so some nurses became involved in campaigns for social justice. One such nurse, Emma Goldman, risked prosecution and imprisonment to campaign for better lives for America's burgeoning working class in the early twentieth century.

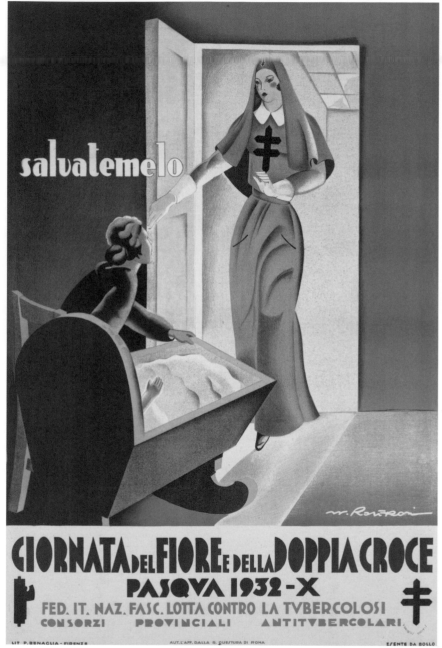

salvatemelo

GIORNATA DEL FIORE E DELLA DOPPIA CROCE
PASQVA 1932-X
FED. IT. NAZ. FASC. LOTTA CONTRO LA TVBERCOLOSI
CONSORZI   PROVINCIALI   ANTITVBERCOLARI

Above:

*A mother appeals to a TB nurse to save her son from
tuberculosis in this Italian anti-TB propaganda
poster. In the early twentieth century tuberculosis was
a leading cause of death in the USA and Europe, and
governments sought to increase public awareness with
propaganda posters like this.*

THE FIGHT AGAINST TUBERCULOSIS

Tuberculosis (TB) nursing developed in the USA
from the early part of the nineteenth century. Ellen
LaMotte, who worked as a TB nurse in Baltimore
just before the First World War, commented on the
independence of such nurses and on the continuity
of their practice. While patients might change
physicians frequently during the course of TB, the
same nurse stayed with them, visiting them on a
regular basis and giving advice on the need for good
diet, cleanliness, and fresh air.

In the late nineteenth and early twentieth centuries, TB was known as the "white plague." Many
thousands of people were affected, and significant numbers died. Thousands of nurses all over
the world worked with TB patients. When
patients were admitted to sanatoria, nurses were
there to care for them, making sure that they
received the rich diet that could help them
combat the wasting effects of the disease, and
rest, exercise, and fresh air in the right quanti-
ties. They also administered the treatments doctors prescribed. Some of these could be quite
"heroic" and included the deliberate surgical collapse of a lung to eradicate the TB bacillus.
Nurses offered comfort, care, and life-saving
attention to patients during these experiences.

Many patients were unable to overcome TB. In the
early twentieth century, nurses were sometimes the
only people who stayed with these distressed individuals, supporting them as they died. Death could
be slow and lingering, or it could be sudden and
dramatic, as when a patient suffered from a fatal
haemoptysis—a sudden, massive bleed from the
lungs. It took immense courage for nurses to
comfort patients during such events, particularly
in the era before antibiotics. Many nurses contracted TB and some died from the disease.

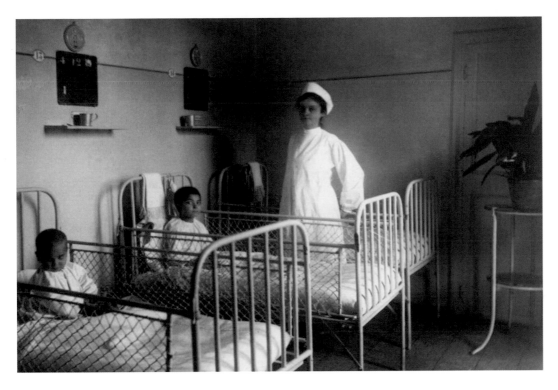

THE FIGHT AGAINST MALARIA

Human beings have suffered from malaria for tens of thousands of years. The protozoan causing the disease was discovered in 1880, and the link to the mosquito in 1898. However, it was only during the twentieth century that a deeper understanding of the disease enabled individuals to protect themselves. Now, for the first time, travelers to hot climates began to wear protective clothing and to sleep under mosquito netting, and campaigns were launched to eradicate mosquitoes from many parts of the world by destroying their habitats. The first effective treatment was the drug quinine, obtained from the bark of the cinchona tree. Although cinchona bark had been available for centuries, the effective use of quinine was relatively new.

Nursing those suffering from malaria was a daunting task. Patients experienced desperately high fevers, joint pains, vomiting, and anemia, and required total care. As well as caring for those with the disease, many nurses, such as Anna Fraentzel-Celli, also turned their attention to preventive work.

Anna Fraentzel-Celli (1878–1958)

Trained as a nurse in Hamburg, Germany, in the late nineteenth century, Anna Fraentzel married the influential Italian public health doctor, Angelo Celli, in 1899 and became closely involved in his work controlling malaria in the Agro Romano—the countryside outside Rome, Italy. Anna visited many villages, advising residents on how to avoid contracting the disease, and distributed quinine, which was the only effective treatment at the time. She also established a system of "auxiliary health visitors" and founded small country schools. Passionate about her work, she once wrote to a friend:

"For my own account, I have only one aim in my life, to do what little I can to fight malaria. But I repeat, I want to go where even a dog would hesitate to go, to show people that it is possible to live and work even in those areas which are most infected with malaria."

In the early twentieth century Anna established a School of Nursing in Rome. She was a remarkable woman who influenced Italian health policy at the highest levels.

NURSING IN REMOTE AREAS

For people living outside cities, even in densely populated parts of Europe, good nursing care was not always easy to come by. In other parts of the world, as exploration and colonization took hold, populations became scattered. Many colonial societies took trained doctors and nurses with them on their expeditions to establish new communities, but as these communities became more and more thinly spread, need began to outstrip supply. At first, these communities coped without expert nursing care, caring for each other as best they could and trusting to the knowledge of their more experienced members. But eventually this was not enough.

The establishment of nursing services in these areas developed gradually and in an ad hoc way. The need was usually first recognized by one individual, who established a service as a philanthropic venture, then campaigned for funds. In most countries, it was some time before national and local governments caught up with pioneering individuals and placed nursing services on a formal footing. This meant that there was a long period during which intrepid nurses worked in very remote areas with no immediate medical support. Their independence and autonomy were extraordinary, and they demonstrated great skill and determination.

The Frontier Nursing Service in the USA

The speed with which the North American continent was colonized in the nineteenth and twentieth centuries was quite remarkable. Migration from the overcrowded cities of the eastern USA to new lands "out west" continued for many decades, and as families eager to start a new life traveled outward from the railroads and other lines of communication, they moved farther and farther away from established medical and nursing services. Very little is known about how health care was brought to most of these vast underpopulated areas during the first decades of the twentieth century. However, thanks to the work of an intrepid American woman named Mary Breckinridge we do have information on one place that was helped and supported during those adventurous times.

Mary Breckinridge (1881–1965)

An extraordinary, energetic woman, Mary Breckinridge was born in 1881, and spent much of her childhood in Washington, where her father represented Arkansas in the US Congress. Much of her education was received at the hands of private governesses and tutors, though she also spent three years at finishing schools in Lausanne, Switzerland, and Stamford, Connecticut. She was said to have been a dazzling and beautiful young woman who loved to dance all night, but her glittering and privileged youth gave way to a heartbreaking adulthood. In November 1904 she married Henry Ruffner Morrison, but he died only a few months later of appendicitis. Three years after this, Mary

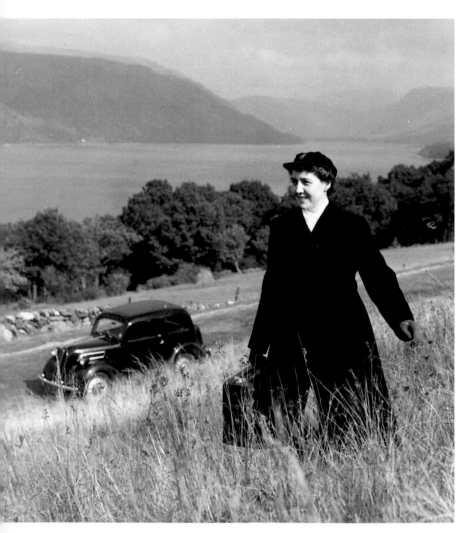

entered the training school at St Luke's Hospital in New York. After graduation, she spent a year caring for her sick mother.

In 1912 she married her second husband and moved to the remote mountain village of Eureka Springs, Arkansas, where she had two children. Her daughter, Polly, lived for only six hours, and her son, Clifton, died of an abdominal infection at the age of four. Soon after his death, Mary and her husband divorced. It was undoubtedly these experiences that inspired Mary to found the Frontier Nursing Service in 1925. She always believed that her son would have survived if only he had had access to good medical care—at the time, Eureka was many miles from the nearest hospital. The experience of losing her children had a profound effect on her, especially when she realized that many families living in poverty in remote parts of the USA had no access to health care of any kind.

Mary decided to establish an experimental rural nursing service in Leslie County, one of the most remote parts of the Appalachian region of Kentucky. She located her district clinics so that no one was far from help, and staffed them with nurse-midwives whose scope of practice was quite extraordinary, ranging from pulling teeth and delivering babies to offering basic advice on hygiene and health education.

One of the earliest clinics was established at Hyden. To reach it, new nurses had to travel from Lexington to Krypton by train, disembark in a siding and then ride on horseback for about 30 miles, traveling along narrow paths and fording rivers en route. They were told to have at least five riding lessons before beginning the journey to their new posting. Many of the cases they visited were childbirth emergencies. In the remote wilds of Kentucky, dealing with a miscarriage or a woman convulsing with eclampsia was an unnerving experience, particularly when it could take a doctor many hours to arrive. In 1952, Mary published the story of the Frontier Nursing Service in a partly autobiographical book, *Wide Neighborhoods*, which brought some welcome publicity.

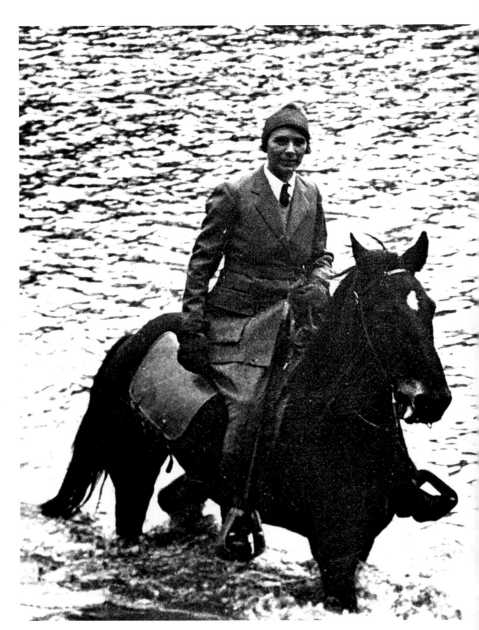

Mary Breckinridge died at the age of eighty-five and continued to work until the day before her death. In the 1960s the Appalachian Mountains were recognized as a region of poverty and designated to receive state aid. By the 1980s Leslie County was no longer the unreachable area nurses had ridden into on horseback in the 1920s. It was now served by fast highways and high-tech medical services.

Above:

Photograph from the Royal College of Nursing Archives, UK, believed to be of a member of the Frontier Nursing Service, Kentucky, USA.

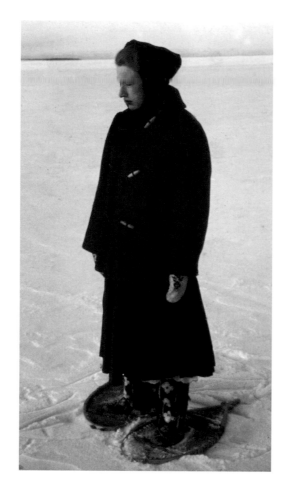

Right:

Susan Brocklehurst (née Engels) worked as a Grenfell nurse in the 1950s. This photograph was taken after her marriage to Grenfell doctor, John Brocklehurst. She is pregnant with her first child, who was later to be delivered by one of her Grenfell nurse-midwife colleagues.

Red Cross Outposts in Canada

After the First World War, the Canadian Red Cross developed outposts in the remotest parts of Canada. Nursing stations were established in small far-northern communities such as Wilberforce, Atikokan, and Coe Hill, where nurses lived and worked assisted only by housekeepers. The work was remarkably broad-ranging. In addition to public health duties such as immunizations and child welfare visits, these nurses, isolated as they were from medical assistance, delivered hundreds of babies, performed surgery under anesthetic, and extracted teeth.

Louise Flach de Kiriline Lawrence (1894–1992)

Born in Sweden, Louise Flach de Kiriline Lawrence undertook her nurse training during the First World War. Her husband, a Russian-born military officer, went missing after the Russian Revolution of 1917. After a long and fruitless search for him, Louise decided to emigrate to Canada. Once there, she devoted her life to outpost nursing. She joined the Red Cross and was posted to the tiny, remote, French Canadian settlement of Bonfield, where she spent many years caring virtually single-handedly for the health of the community.

The Grenfell Mission Nurses in Newfoundland and Labrador

The health care of Labrador (in those days a British territory) was transformed when Wilfred Grenfell, a young doctor working for the British Royal National Mission to Deep Sea Fishermen, first landed on the coast there in 1892. Realizing that the inhabitants of this remote and wild part of the world had no access to medical care of any kind, Grenfell decided to establish a mission to offer them help. His motives were deeply religious.

Grenfell founded nursing stations throughout Newfoundland and Labrador. In each, a single nurse would work with a housekeeper, caring for a widely scattered community, offering health advice, immunizations and emergency treatment, caring for patients with infectious or chronic diseases, and providing both routine and emergency maternity care. The scope of duties for these nurses was vast. Practicing alone, with only untrained staff as assistants, they did some amazing work. Doctors and nurses moved up and down the coast in the summer on mission boats such as the converted fishing schooner *Maraval*, which carried X-ray machines, and operating theaters where surgery could be performed. Eventually, the mission grew into a large organization known as the International Grenfell Association. Health services in Labrador and Newfoundland were built on the foundations it had created.

Much of our knowledge of these adventurous times in Newfoundland and Labrador comes from the fascinating memoirs of one Grenfell nurse called Lesley Diack, who wrote about some of her experiences there.

Lesley Diack

After serving as an Army Nursing Sister in the Second World War, Lesley, who was clearly a woman who thrived on adventure, signed up for the Grenfell Mission in 1948.

The work was unpredictable. At some times, Lesley's ward could be quite empty; at others it was full of seriously ill patients who needed constant care. One particularly stressful aspect of the job was the frequent arrival of expectant mothers at the station. It was impossible to predict just when they would give birth, and sometimes several babies would be delivered on successive nights, meaning no sleep for the nurse.

The seasons on the Labrador coast were harsh and extreme. In winter, the sea froze and airplanes could land on the ice. It was also possible to travel overland by dog-team, which meant that emergency patients could be transported rapidly to hospital. In the spring, however, when the ice began to thaw, conditions could be extremely difficult, since any traveling had to be done partly on foot, and partly by canoe, navigating across bogs and semi-thawed lakes. In summer, transport was by boat, but in the fall, as storms lashed the coast and the ice began to form once more, travel could become impossible, and nurses were often trapped in their stations for days or weeks at a time.

Lesley treated many sick people and delivered dozens of babies during her first three years at the mission. In Forteau, she was the only trained health professional and, as it was often impossible for specialist help to reach her, she had to take on the role of physician, surgeon, obstetrician, and dentist. She was also the only public health worker for miles around, visiting families throughout her district to give immunizations, vitamins, antenatal advice and support. When epidemics broke out, her hospital would be crowded with small, very sick children. One recurrent emergency was the mauling of young children by husky dogs. Lesley describes one such case—a little girl who was brought into the hospital:

"Most of her scalp had been torn off, but it was still partially attached with just sufficient blood supply to enable it to be put back again…Sixteen stitches were required for the scalp alone."

One of Lesley's most stressful operations was the lancing of an abscess in the jaw of a very small boy, which she had to perform by following verbal instructions over the radio-transmitter from the doctor in the next community. On another occasion, she had to carry out emergency surgery on a woman whose afterbirth had failed to be delivered. She did the procedure, while at the same time directing her untrained assistant, who was giving the anesthetic. The operation was a success and the mother lived.

Lesley's work was often grueling, but her love of the beautiful Labrador landscapes, her sense of the great importance of her work, and the kindness and wonderful hospitality of the local people helped her through.

Below:
A group of Grenfell staff taking a break. Lesley Diack is on the left of this photograph. Her dog, Brutus, is pictured in the foreground.

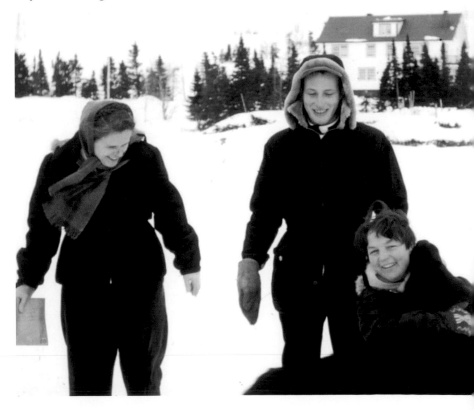

Bush Nursing in Australia

There are few places in the world more remote than parts of Australia. "Bush nursing" services began to emerge after 1910, initially serving populations within 50 miles of cities—even at this distance there were few medical services and no help for those who became ill. The formation of Bush Nursing Associations was the result of the efforts of philanthropic ladies, who recognized the risks taken by those who lived outside cities. The earliest Bush Nursing Association was formed in Melbourne, Victoria, in September 1910, and was largely the work of Rachel Ward, wife of Australia's Governor-General, the Earl of Dudley.

Organizing committees in rural areas raised funds and then applied to the association for a qualified nurse. The nurse's salary continued to be paid by money raised locally, which meant that there was a close and loyal relationship between the nurse and the community she served. First to apply were the inhabitants of Beech Forest, at the end of a narrow gauge railway line that had been built mainly to serve the thriving timber trade. They appointed a nurse called Mary Thompson, who was already known in the area for her compassion and expertise. Stories had been told of how she had nursed a woman in nearby Nhill through pneumonia, and had managed to save the woman's life by her constant attention. It was also known that she had demanded no fee for this work. Before going to Beech Forest, Mary spent two weeks learning from experienced district nurses in Melbourne. Ironically, her first patient was a man who had protested against the employment of a nurse—a railway construction supervisor who suffered from concussion after an accident.

By 1912 there were six bush nursing centers in Victoria, four in New South Wales, and one in Tasmania. From these small beginnings, the bush nursing service was to spread across Australia.

The normal uniform of the bush nurses in Victoria consisted of pale gray dresses and white aprons, collars, and cuffs. However, nurses usually wore a riding habit, oilskins, and strong boots while on duty, because of the long distances to be traveled on horseback. They carried their equipment in a portmanteau or saddlebags, taking with them to visits: syringes and needles; medications and ointments; temperature charts; dressings; sheets; catheters; bedpans; feeding cups; surgical needles, scissors and thread; and many other pieces of equipment. They did not travel light and could not have done their work as efficiently as they did without some form of transport. They usually rode to their visits on horseback. The bulk of their work involved delivering babies; giving emergency care to accident victims; attending the sick—who were often suffering from infectious diseases; caring for patients following surgery; and doing child-health checks in schools. Their emergency and maternity patients could sometimes only be reached after dramatic and difficult nighttime journeys.

Below:

Photograph of nurse and baby Andrew John taken on a survey trip carried out in 1927 by Dr J.A. Barker and Dr John Simpson for the Flying Doctor Service.

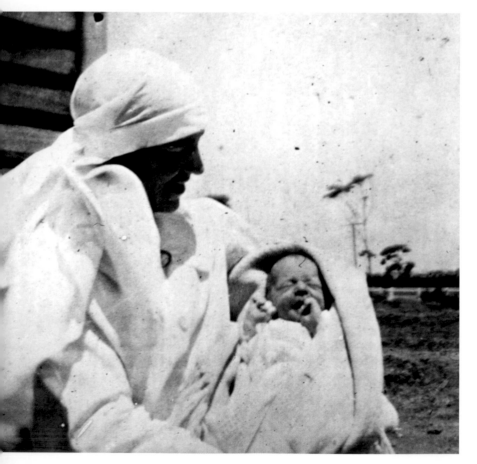

Australia's Flying Nurses

The Australian Flying Doctor Service has an interesting link with the Bush Nursing movement. The man who is credited with founding the service, Reverend John Flynn, had his first posting as a Home Missionary in Beech Forest in 1903, and, although he left before the appointment of Mary Thompson, his association with this early pioneering community seems a remarkable coincidence. In 1914, he founded the Australian Inland Mission, which went on to establish "hostels" in remote areas. These were later renamed "nursing homes," and each was staffed by two nursing sisters.

It is believed that Flynn may have come up with the idea of the Flying Doctor Service as early as 1911, but the first written mention of the idea doesn't appear until a letter he wrote to the mission's journal, the *Inlander*, in 1918. In the 1920s, with the development of the wireless radio, homesteads in remote parts of Australia could maintain contact with medical services and receive verbal advice. Then in 1927, charitable funds were made available for an experimental Flying Doctor service in Cloncurry, Queensland. The first flight was to a bush Nursing Center at remote Julia Creek. Eventually, from these small beginnings, the Royal Flying Doctor Service was to emerge. Sections were formed in all Australian states.

From the first, nurses had an important role in the service, preparing dangerously ill and unstable patients for arduous journeys, and often traveling with them from remote outback areas to hospitals during flights that could take several hours. Over a period of many decades, the service became increasingly sophisticated, with the availability of portable onboard life-support equipment. This meant that nurses themselves also had to have a sophisticated approach to the care of their patients, understanding how to use the latest technology, and being capable of reacting to any emergency.

Plunket Nurses in New Zealand

In New Zealand, shocked by the appalling infant death rates at the turn of the century, Dr Frederick Truby King was driven to inaugurate several public health nursing schemes. The most famous of these was The Plunket Society, founded in 1907 and named after Victoria Plunket, the wife of New Zealand's then Governor-General. Plunket nurses were trained at the society's center in Dunedin to visit homes and give public health advice to mothers. They visited women from all social classes in all parts of New Zealand, and often formed close friendships with the mothers they helped, becoming highly respected figures in their local communities. This scheme inspired the development of the similarly run Mothercraft Training Society in Britain in 1918.

Working as a public health nurse in New Zealand was challenging. In the "back-blocks"—the remotest parts of the country—nurses worked alone offering total care to their patients.

Below:
Flight Nurse Briody Main and ambulance officers from the Queensland Ambulance Service prepare a stretcher to be flown from Cairns to Townsville Hospital on an aircraft of the Royal Flying Doctor Service.

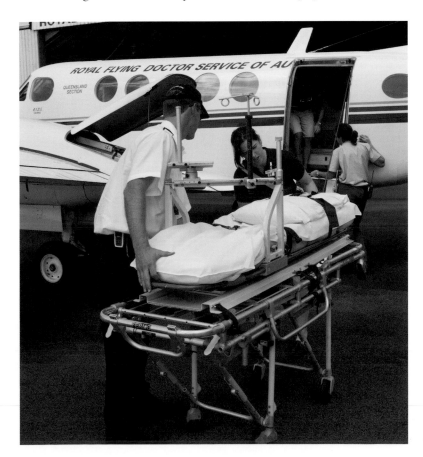

THE CAMPAIGN FOR BIRTH CONTROL

In the early twentieth century, a combination of widespread poverty and the opening-up of a new motivation among women to control their own lives led to a desire for family limitation. Women had very few birth control methods at their disposal, relying mainly on the oldest method of contraception: *coitus interruptus* (interrupted intercourse). Early barrier methods such as condoms and cervical caps were difficult to use and were not widely known, and women often turned to desperate measures such as the use of "abortifacients" (herbal and chemical substances that were used to induce miscarriage), which were highly dangerous.

Society in those times was still highly patriarchal and heavily influenced by a powerful institutional church that was adamantly opposed to birth control, seeing it as a subversion of God's laws. It was not until the second decade of that century that women (and some men) began to campaign for effective and safe contraception.

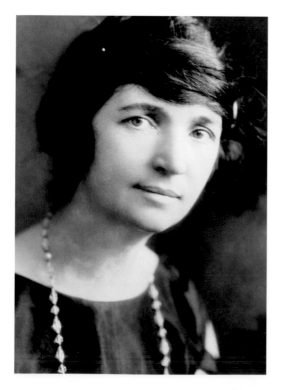

Right:

Margaret Sanger trained as a nurse in White Plains. She spent most of her life campaigning for women's right to birth control.

Margaret Sanger (1879–1966)

Born Margaret Higgins in Corning, New York, Margaret Sanger was to become one of the most influential—and controversial—campaigners for birth control in the world. Her work was driven, in part, by her feelings about her own mother's tragic life and death. Anne Higgins, a committed Roman Catholic, had eighteen pregnancies, eleven of which resulted in live births. Margaret was her sixth child. During her youth, Margaret spent a lot of her time caring for her younger siblings, but when she went to college her older sisters paid her tuition fees for two years. When the money ran out, Margaret came home to care for her mother, who was dying of TB and cervical cancer. Following this experience, she enrolled in nurse training in White Plains.

In 1902, Margaret married an architect, William Sanger. She had developed TB as a result of caring for her mother, and she and her husband went to live in Saranac in the Adirondack Mountains in the belief that the mountain air would help cure her condition. The move was successful, and Margaret regained her health. She gave birth to her first son in 1903.

Years later, the family moved to New York City, where Margaret worked as a nurse in the deprived East Side of Manhattan. Already interested in sexuality and birth control, she began to write a column for the *New York Call* entitled "What Every Girl Should Know." She also distributed a pamphlet called *Family Limitation*. At that time, US law stated that the publication and distribution of this type of material was obscene and therefore illegal. Margaret's counterargument was that the state made such laws not in the interests of the people, but in order that State and Church could enforce control over women's lives.

While working on the Lower East Side, Margaret had an experience that increased her determination to campaign for birth control. She was called to the house of a woman named Sadie Sachs, who was dangerously ill following an illegal abortion. Sadie had asked her doctor for advice on how to prevent another pregnancy—he had simply told her to abstain from sexual intercourse. Months later, Margaret was once again called to Sadie's apartment, to find that her patient had died while trying to induce another abortion. In 1914, Margaret began to publish *The Woman Rebel*, a newsletter promoting contraception. She was prosecuted for breaking the US obscenity laws, but fled to England under a false name. On her return to New York she opened her first birth control clinic, but it was closed down by the authorities, and Margaret served a thirty-day prison sentence. In 1916, Margaret published *What Every Girl Should Know*, a book on female sexuality and birth control that was to be highly influential.

The breakthrough came in 1923, when Margaret discovered a loophole in the law, and was able to open the first legal birth control clinic in the USA, which was secretly funded by John D. Rockefeller. Over the next few decades, she lectured in public halls throughout the USA, and spoke at international academic conferences about her work. She formed the National Committee on Federal Legislation for Birth Control, and was its president until, in 1937, many states legalized birth control. In that year, Margaret was made Chair of the Birth Control Council of America. She was to serve on a number of national and international councils during the course of her life and published several books, including *Motherhood in Bondage*, a compilation of letters sent to her by women desperate for information on birth control. Margaret Sanger died at the age of eighty-six, having had a massive influence on thinking about both freedom of speech and the right of women to control their own reproduction.

Marie Stopes (1880–1958)

When Margaret Sanger fled to England in 1915, she met a young scientist, Marie Stopes. Margaret had a great influence on Marie, who was herself to become a birth control campaigner.

An accomplished scientist with two doctorates, Marie married Humphrey Vernon Roe in 1918, and her husband helped fund the publication of her

book, *Married Love*, which offered frank, clear advice on family planning. It became a bestseller, and was followed by several other books and pamphlets on contraception and family life. In 1921, Marie opened the Mother's Clinic in the poverty-stricken London neighborhood of Upper Holloway. Staffed by nurses and one female doctor, the clinic offered advice to women and fitted vaginal caps, sparking a revolution in health care. Marie Stopes clinics eventually opened throughout Britain, and also in South Africa, Australia, and New Zealand.

Below:
Scientist Marie Stopes had an important influence on birth control in the UK. Her first clinic was established in Upper Holloway, London.

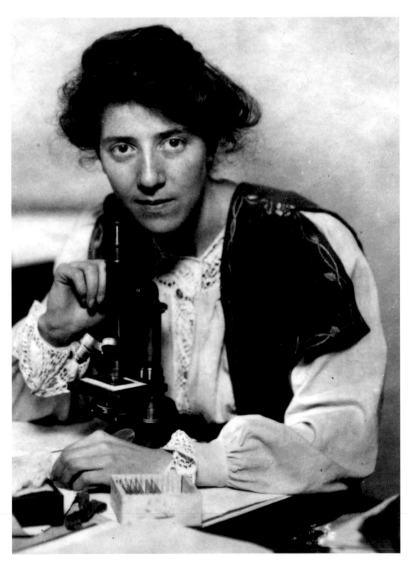

A DEVELOPING PROFESSION

Nursing itself was changing in two important ways. First, it was freeing itself from its image as a profession for women only. In every era, from the "Camillians" of the sixteenth century to the orderlies of the First World War military hospitals, men had worked as carers. After the Second World War, throughout the developed world, it was increasingly seen as right that men should be admitted to formal nurse training schools. Although few recruitment drives were directed deliberately at the male population, the heads of nurse training schools were no longer viewing nursing as an exclusively female occupation, and from the mid-century onward men entered nurse training schools in greater numbers.

Secondly, nurses were also changing their perceptions of what it took to become a "trained nurse." Indeed, toward the end of the century, the word "training" was becoming much less popular than "education." In the USA, Adelaide Nutting blazed the trail for university nurse-academics by becoming the first Professor of Nursing in the world. In other countries, nursing education was much slower to move into universities. In Britain, for example, the process was not complete until the last few years of the twentieth century. Yet in all parts of the world, nursing was coming to be seen as a "discipline" in its own right.

Adelaide Nutting (1858–1948)

In 1907, Adelaide Nutting became the first Professor of Nursing in the world, when she accepted the offer of a Chair at Teachers College, Columbia University, New York. By 1910, she had enlarged her department of Household Administration and had renamed it the Department of Nursing and Health. Before moving to New York, Adelaide had been Superintendent of Nurses at the Johns Hopkins Hospital Training School in Baltimore for sixteen years. The move to Teachers College enabled her to develop nursing as a discipline in its own right, with its own knowledge base.

NURSING DEVELOPS AS A DISCIPLINE

During the twentieth century, nursing education curricula were developed all over the world. Britain was one of the earliest countries to gain a standard national syllabus, which was designed to be taught in all hospital training schools. The newly founded General Nursing Council established a state examination for nurses in the early 1920s.

Although its education was formalized at quite an early date, the nursing profession in Britain was slow to move its "trainees" into universities and make them fully fledged "students." One of the earliest experimental university programs was developed in 1959 at the University of Manchester by public health professor, Colin Fraser Brockington. This became a degree in 1969. At this time, several universities began to develop programs for nurses, and by 1997 all nurse education had moved into universities.

Jean McFarlane (1926–)

Born in Cardiff, South Wales, Jean McFarlane spent her childhood in a busy professional household. Her father, qualified in both medicine and dentistry, was a practicing dentist. His interest in public health and his enthusiasm for health care were to be an enduring influence on her. As a teenager Jean assisted him in administering anesthetics to his patients and then in helping her mother "revive" these patients with a "cup of Mrs Mac's coffee."

After spending a year studying chemistry, Jean decided to enter the nursing profession—in spite of attempts by her teachers and peers to dissuade her. In 1947, she entered nurse training at St Bartholomew's School of Nursing, London. Her experience of acute hospital care convinced her that "prevention was better than cure." It was in the community, she felt, that the greatest differences could be made to people's lives, so she decided to enter health visiting.

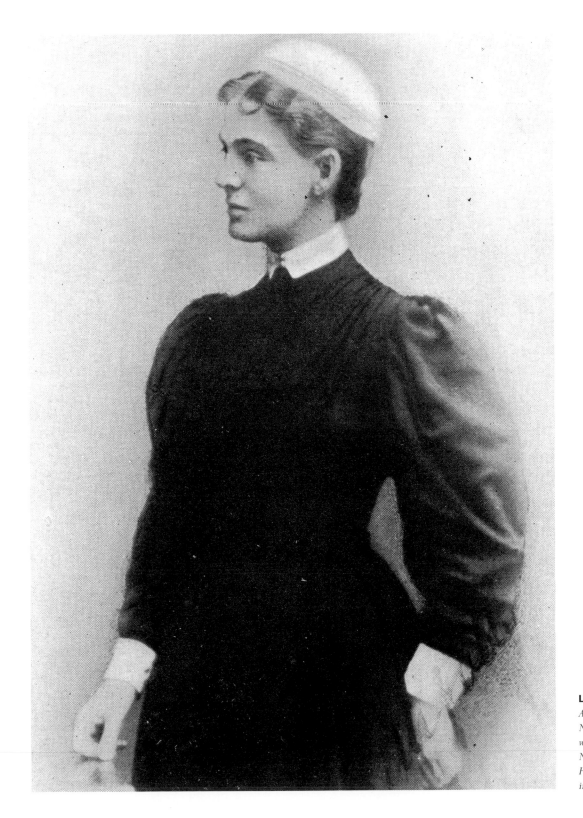

Left:
*A photograph of Adelaide
Nutting, taken when she
was Superintendent of
Nurses at Johns Hopkins
Hospital Training School
in Baltimore.*

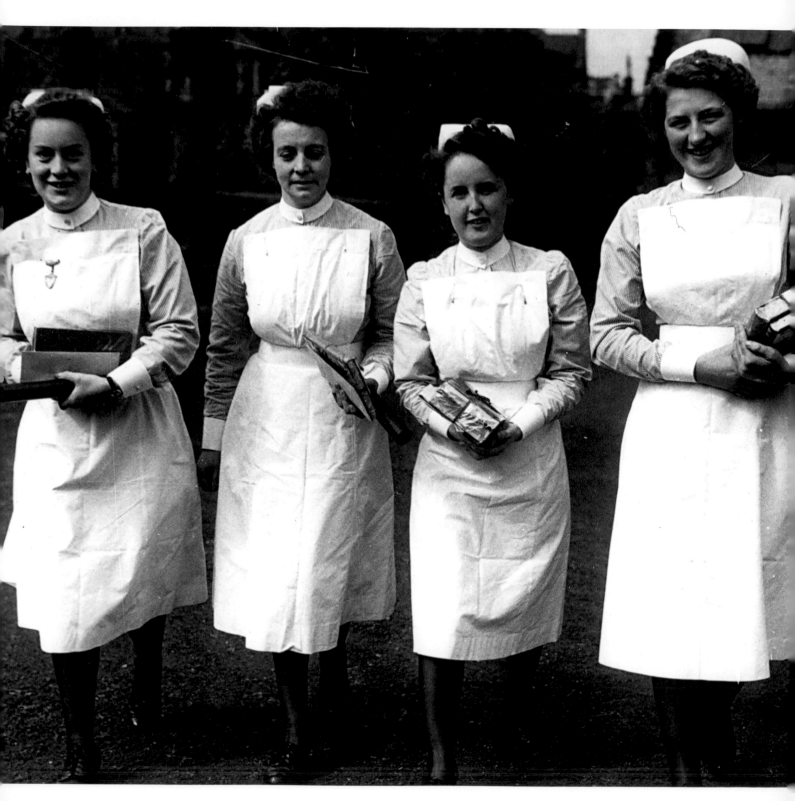

In 1966, Jean was invited to lead the Study of Nursing Care project at the Royal College of Nursing (RCN), which led to a series of important new publications about nursing care. Running through the series was a strong affirmation of the value of nursing work.

After spending a year as Director of Education at the RCN, Jean was invited to become the head of the Nursing Section at the University of Manchester. In 1969, the Bachelor of Nursing degree was established there—the first degree in the UK to make nursing its primary focus of study. The University of Manchester rapidly became the center of the concept of the Nursing Process, attracting tutors and practitioners from all over the UK. In 1973, a Department of Nursing was established at the university, and in 1974 Jean became the first Professor of Nursing in England. It was not until 2009 that legislation was passed to raise all British nursing education to degree level.

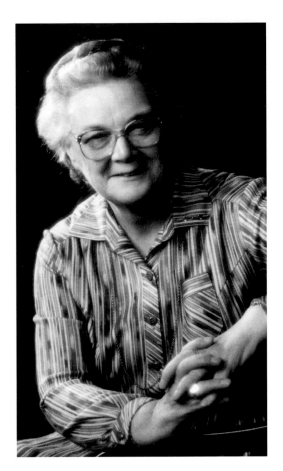

Left:
Jean McFarlane, the first Professor of Nursing in England. In 1979 she became Baroness McFarlane of Llandaff, in acknowledgment of her services to the nursing profession and in particular her role on the Royal Commission on the National Health Service. She devoted her life to developing nursing as a discipline, always keeping the needs of patients at the center of her field of vision.

Opposite:
Four British student nurses from the mid-twentieth century.

"They told me if you've got any brains you have a responsibility to use them, and they didn't think I'd use brains in nursing, and—it's funny—I've found that nursing has used all the intelligence I've got."

Jean McFarlane

Quoted in a 2003 interview

NURSING THEORIES AND MODELS

In the second half of the twentieth century the USA saw the emergence of a new and vibrant movement that would seek to define nursing and study it in depth. For the first time, influential university-based nurses developed detailed theories and models that offered insight into the work they were doing. This work was important because it defined nursing as a discipline in its own right. It also staked a number of claims for the nursing profession: for example, the claim that nursing was very different from medicine, and something that must be done alongside (but not under the direction of) medical work in order to ensure the best outcome for the patient. These theories and models were an assertion that there were things that only a nurse could do and understand.

Virginia Henderson (1897–1996)

One of the most influential of nursing theorists, Virginia Henderson was born in 1897 and spent much of her childhood in Missouri. She trained at the Army School of Nursing in Washington D.C. during the First World War. She worked as a staff nurse at the Henry Street Settlement (see page 75) upon qualification in 1921. From 1922 to 1927, she worked at the Norfolk Protestant Hospital in Virginia before studying for her Bachelor of Science and Master of Arts degrees at Teachers College, Columbia University. In 1930, she returned to Teachers College, and taught the theory and practice of nursing there for several years.

Virginia Henderson coauthored an important textbook with Bertha Harmer entitled *Textbook of the Principles and Practice of Nursing*. In 1955, Virginia edited the fifth edition of this book, adding her own definition of nursing, which was to become highly influential.

Virginia Henderson was clearly able to tap into a rich and vibrant history of thinking and reflection about the nature of nursing practice. An eloquent teacher and wonderfully clear writer, she was also able to translate these ideas into readable and usable texts for nurses. Her pamphlet, *Basic Principles of Nursing Care*, was written for the International Council of Nurses in 1960 and was translated into more than twenty languages. Her most famous book, *The Nature of Nursing*, was published in 1966 and had an incalculable influence on nurse-education throughout the world. In it, she explained how nurses worked by enabling their patients to meet a range of needs, and reiterated her world-famous definition of nursing:

"The unique function of the nurse is to assist the individual, sick or well, in the performance of those activities contributing to health or its recovery (or to a peaceful death) that he would perform unaided if he had the necessary strength, will or knowledge. And to do this in such a way as to help him gain independence as rapidly as possible. This aspect of her work, this part of her function, she initiates and controls; of this she is the master."

Virginia's work blazed the trail for other nurse theorists who designed a range of models to explain the complexity of nursing work. From Sister Callista Roy, who defined nursing as a means by which the nurse helped the patient to "adapt" to

> *"The unique function of the nurse is to assist the individual, sick or well, in the performance of those activities contributing to health or its recovery."*
>
> Virginia Henderson
>
> *Extract from* The Nature of Nursing *(1966)*

the stresses that had made him ill, to Dorothea Orem, who defined illness as a deficit in "self-care," and the nurse as the person who would enable the person to become independent again, these theorists thrived in the atmosphere of questioning and debate that was fostered by university nursing departments in the middle decades of the twentieth century.

Patricia Benner

A Professor in the Department of Physiological Nursing in the School of Nursing at the University of California, San Francisco, Patricia Benner developed her theory of nursing expertise during the 1980s. Her book, *From Novice to Expert*, became a classic of nursing literature. For Benner, the expert nurse was one who could accurately and quickly assess a patient's needs, take action in a way that would help improve the patient's condition (directly involving the patient in these processes, where possible), and achieve a positive outcome that could be carefully monitored. Often, expertise seemed a mysterious process because so much judgment and decision-making was taking place so rapidly in the mind of the nurse—invisible to the outside observer.

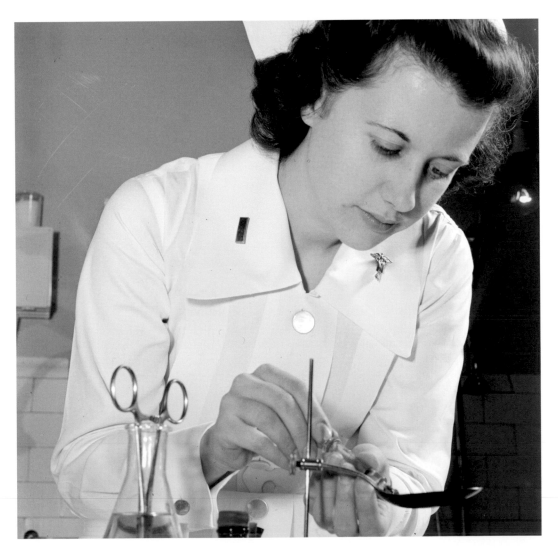

Left:

In the mid-twentieth century, nurse training had a strong scientific component and experimental lab-work was employed to enable students to better understand physiological processes and the actions of chemically based drugs. In this photograph a student nurse in Washington D.C., close to qualification, performs an experiment in a laboratory setting.

NURSING CARE
AND GLOBAL HEALTH

Nurses made important contributions to global health. Through charitable organizations such as Médecins Sans Frontières and Voluntary Services Overseas, many trained nurses offered their valuable services free of charge to aid agencies in deprived and developing parts of the world, or in regions struck by disaster. By making important contributions to public health through immunization and education programs, and caring directly for the sick, these nurses made a positive difference to global health and development.

Nursing at the World Health Organization (WHO)

The World Health Organization (WHO) was established soon after the Second World War as part of an attempt to regenerate the health and welfare of ruined nations. Nurses influenced global health through Nursing Officers, who were appointed to the organization's regional offices. Decades after its formation, WHO declared the breadth and scope of its ambitions by defining health as a state of total physical, mental, and social wellbeing and "not merely the absence of disease." Nurses were at the forefront of its important global public health initiatives, which were ambitious and effective.

Mother Teresa (1910–1997)

Born Agnese Gonxhe Bojaxhiu in Uskub (now Skopje) in Macedonia, Mother Teresa was a Roman Catholic nun who founded the Missionaries of Charity in Calcutta in 1950. She left home at the age of eighteen to become a missionary, first joining the Sisters of Loreto in Rathfarnham, Ireland. Once she had learned English, she moved to Darjeeling in India, to commence the work she had wanted to do since childhood—caring for the poor and sick. Eventually, she abandoned her nun's habit, began to wear a sari, and took Indian citizenship. She started a school in Motijhil, but soon expanded her work to care for anyone who was unwanted and uncared-for—shunned by society. She opened her first Home for the Dying in 1952 in an abandoned Hindu temple in Calcutta, and her first hospital for lepers soon afterward.

The Missionaries of Charity founded soup kitchens, orphanages, and schools as well as hospitals, but among its most important work was the development of specialist centers for the care of the sick. Some journalists and medical writers criticized Teresa's work for its lack of attention to "proper" diagnosis and its emphasis on valuing poverty.

The Missionaries of Charity expanded rapidly throughout Mother Teresa's lifetime, and established centers throughout the world. Mother Teresa became one of the most famous humanitarian workers ever known, and was awarded the Nobel Peace Prize in 1979. She was not a trained nurse, yet by working with and giving opportunities to those who were trained and experienced, she opened up possibilities for them to do important work. She also demonstrated that it was possible for anyone to improve the lives of their fellow human beings by doing what work they could. In a significant way, Mother Teresa, one of the most modern aid-workers, takes the story of nursing "full-circle," back to the ancient and medieval worlds where altruistic individuals took in and cared for those shunned by the rest of society.

Right:
Danish nurse Erna Spohrhanssen working at Albert Schweitzer's hospital village in Lambarene, Gabon (Africa), in 1954.

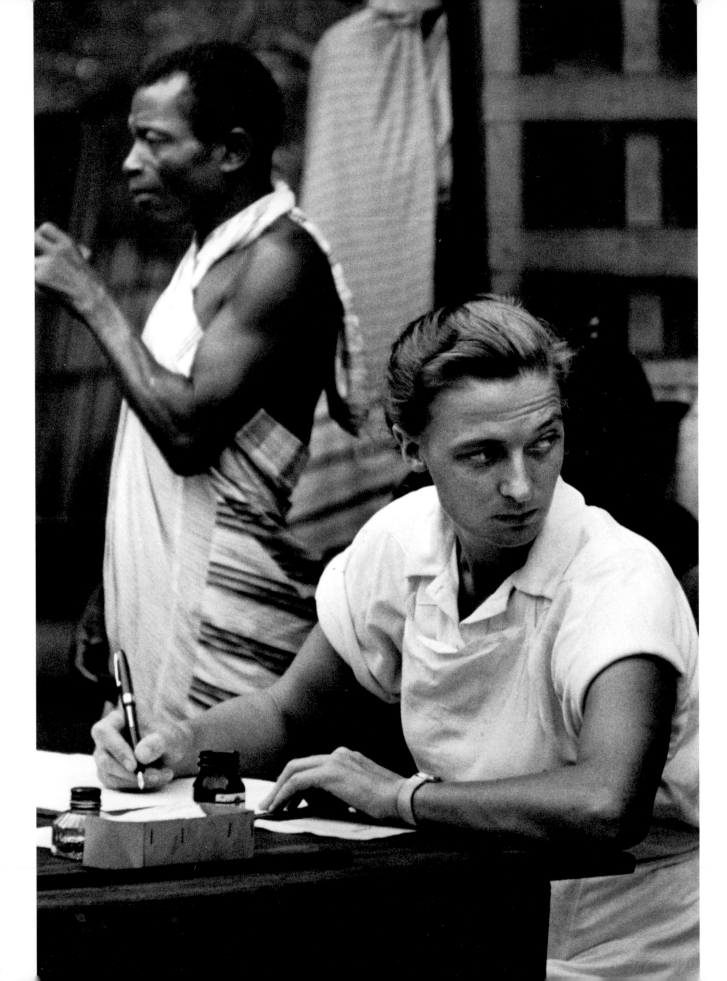

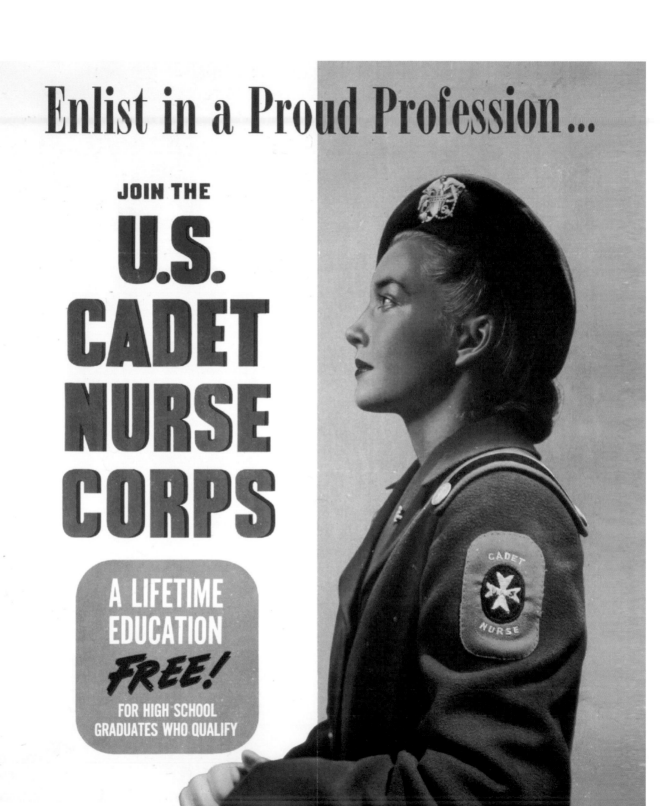

Enlist in a Proud Profession...

JOIN THE

U.S. CADET NURSE CORPS

A LIFETIME EDUCATION *FREE!*
FOR HIGH SCHOOL GRADUATES WHO QUALIFY

Nurses On the Front Line

At the beginning of the twentieth century nurses were learning from the experiences of their colleagues in the preceding century. It had become clear during the Second Boer War (1899–1902) in South Africa that specially trained and experienced nurses were needed to lead those who cared for the war-wounded. The Boer War had taught many important lessons—particularly in relation to the dangers of epidemic diseases for troops who lived and fought closely together. During the war more men had died from disease than from injury. It also illustrated the need to intensify existing public health efforts. So many volunteers, when examined, were found to be "unfit for service" that anxieties were raised about the capacity of the population to defend itself in future wars. Only a small cadre of nurses joined the Royal Army Medical Corps in South Africa, but its members proved their worth and demonstrated the need for an organized nursing service.

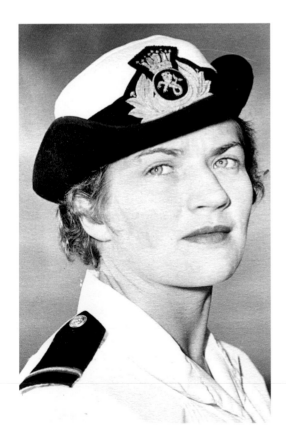

MILITARY NURSING CORPS

As the twentieth century opened, the American Army Nurse Corps was being formed. It was established in 1901, with Jane Delano (see page 57) as its first Superintendent, and developed into one of the most effective elite nursing corps in the world. A year later, in 1902, the British followed with the formation of the Queen Alexandra's Imperial Military Nursing Service. It was from the ranks of organizations such as these that nurses were drawn to serve in the major conflicts of the century.

Left:
A mid-twentieth century British Navy nurse.

Opposite:
A US government recruitment poster from 1943, used as part of a drive to bring more nurses into the armed forces when the Second World War was at its height.

FIRST WORLD WAR (1914–1918)

By the beginning of the First World War, the
membership of Queen Alexandra's Imperial
Military Nursing Service in Britain had grown to
about 300; and the service could call on a number
of "reservists." These numbers expanded rapidly
following the outbreak of war. In addition, the
staffs of general hospitals throughout the country
formed the Territorial Force Nursing Service,
ready to receive the wounded, or go abroad
on active service at just twenty-four hours' notice.
There was, nevertheless, still an acute shortage
of nurses, and thousands of volunteers from
Voluntary Aid Detachments (VADs) were
recruited by military hospitals both at home and
abroad. A great deal of nursing work was done by
these VADs, and by military orderlies, under the
supervision of trained nurses.

The work was arduous and often distressing.
Nurses and their colleagues were caring for men
who had suffered severe mutilating injuries. Many
patients lost one or more limbs or parts of their
faces. To make these injuries worse, the fact that
battles took place over heavily manured farmland
meant that horrific infections such as gas gangrene
and tetanus could take hold very quickly. Nurses
tackled these by giving injections of antitetanus
serum, and by applying antiseptics.

One of the greatest horrors of the war was gas poi-
soning. Both sides used toxic gases, which they
often shot into enemy trenches in the form of "gas
shells." Chlorine and mustard gases had terrible
effects on victims, burning the skin and destroying
the lining of the respiratory tract so that sufferers
were unable to breathe and often died of suffocation. Nurses did all they could to keep these desperately ill and totally dependent men alive, from
giving oxygen and medications to feeding and
offering comfort and care.

The Western Front

On the Allied side, nurses from Britain, France,
Belgium, Australia, New Zealand, Canada, South
Africa, and the USA worked side by side in military hospitals. When a man was wounded on the
Western Front he was taken to his battalion first-
aid post where a first dressing was applied and
morphine was given. He was then conveyed as
quickly as possible, by ambulance, to a casualty
clearing station, where emergency surgery might
be carried out. After this, he was moved "down the
line" by train or canal barge to a base hospital
(many of which were located on the northern
coast of France) and then finally to Britain, where
he would recuperate in an "auxiliary hospital."
Country houses, schools, and public buildings of
all kinds were routinely pressed into service as
hospitals for this purpose, and some men could
find themselves recovering in the splendor of an
English country mansion.

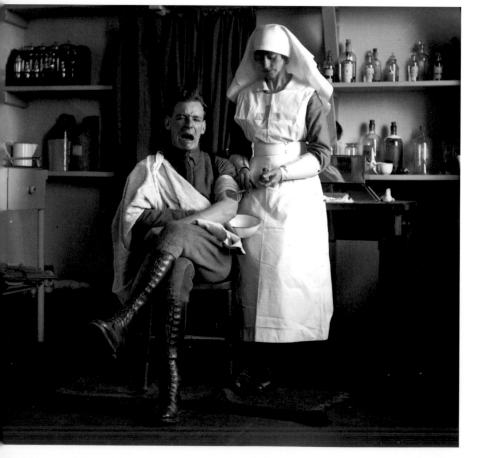

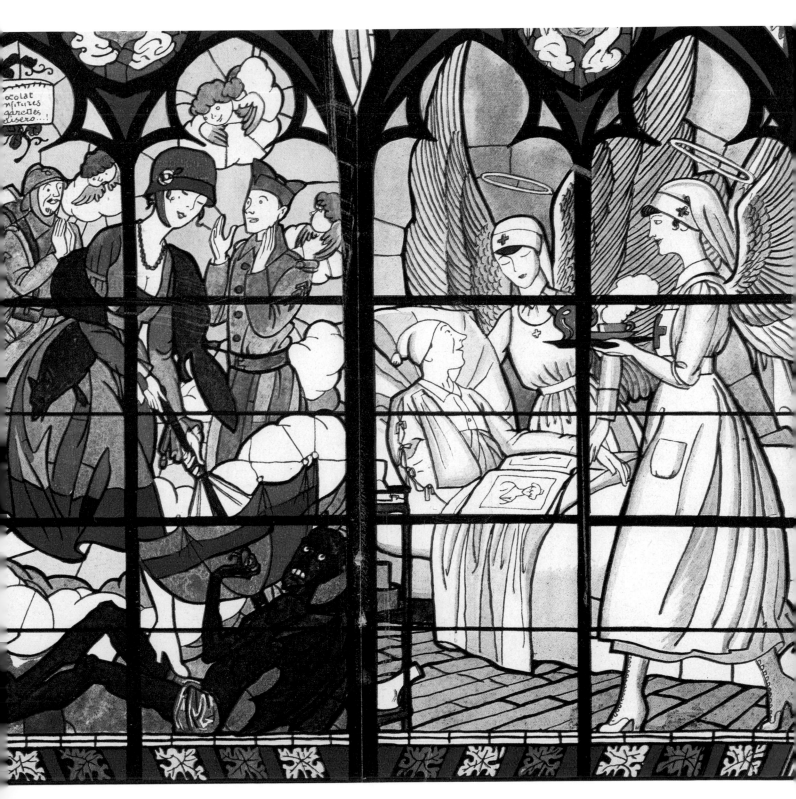

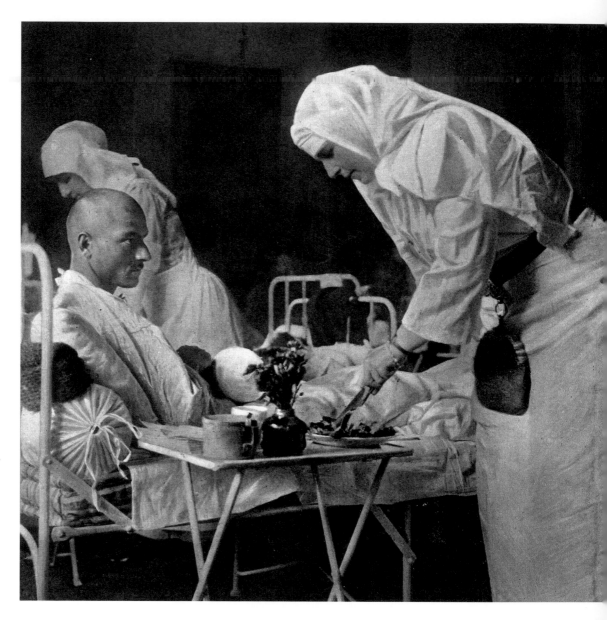

Right:

*Queen Marie of Romania
tends to a wounded soldier
in the Palais Royal of
Bucharest, which was
converted into a hospital.*

Opposite:

*Maud McCarthy was
Matron-in-Chief to the
British Expeditionary Force
in France and Flanders
during the First World War.*

The Eastern Front

On other fronts, care was less clearly organized.
On the Eastern Front, in Russia and Poland,
advances and retreats were so rapid that nurses
worked in "flying columns"—temporary hospitals
that could be uprooted and moved at only a few
hours' notice. Loaded onto wagons, hospital
equipment and supplies could follow an advancing army, or make a rapid escape just ahead of a
retreating one.

In the Eastern Mediterranean, nurses did vital
life-saving work on board hospital ships, on which
the wounded from the Gallipoli peninsula were
transported to hospitals on the Greek island
of Lemnos, or Egypt. And in Salonika, Greece,
nurses cared for patients from the Serbian
campaign, many of whom were desperately ill
with malaria, dysentery, or the notorious
"trench-foot," which resulted from standing in
ice-cold water for days at a time.

Maud McCarthy (1858–1949)

A remarkable, effective nurse, and an exceptional organizer, Maud McCarthy was an extraordinary woman. She was Matron-in-Chief to the British Expeditionary Force in France and Flanders throughout the First World War.

Born Emma Maud McCarthy in Sydney, in 1858, she moved to London in 1891, in order to train as a nurse at the London Hospital. At that time the hospital and training school were under the control of the indomitable Eva Luckes. As a probationer Maud was reported to have been "conscientious" and "exceptionally nice," but lacking in forcefulness. She worked as a ward sister for some time before embarking with a contingent of nurses for South Africa, where she gave distinguished service during the Boer War of 1899–1902. She became a senior member of Britain's newly formed Queen Alexandra's Imperial Military Nursing Service on its formation in 1902, and in 1910 was appointed Principal Matron at the War Office.

When Britain declared war in August 1914, Maud traveled to France with one of the first contingents of nurses. She formed her headquarters at Abbéville, and remained there as Matron-in-Chief, until British forces evacuated the city in March 1918 during the devastating German advance, when she was forced to retreat to Boulogne. Maud took on the responsibility of mobilizing and deploying all the British, Dominion, and American nurses in Northern France during the war, and the effectiveness of the military hospitals on the Western Front was largely due to her skill and organizing ability. She undertook very frequent "tours" of the Western Front casualty clearing stations and base hospitals, personally making sure that the nursing services were up to the required standard, and that they had the support and resources they needed.

After the war, Maud became Matron-in-Chief to the Territorial Force Nursing Service; she retired in 1925. She died in London in 1949, at the age of ninety.

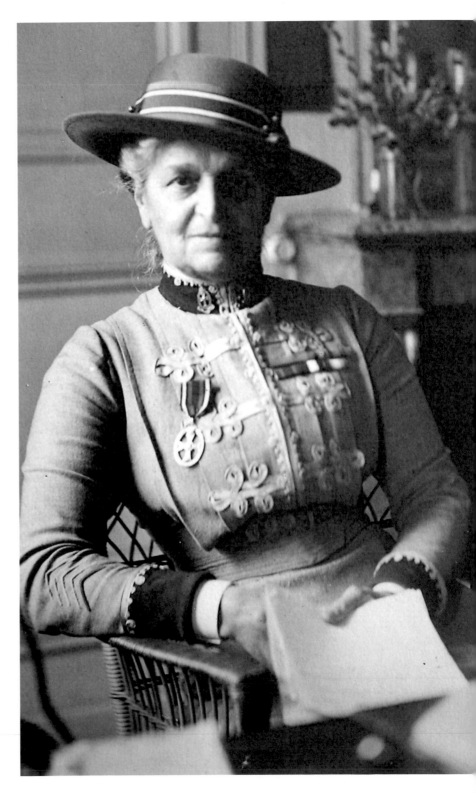

Violetta Thurstan (1879–1978)

When Britain entered the First World War in August 1914, Violetta Thurstan not only offered herself for active service, but went straight to the most dangerous area of the conflict: the Belgian front. In Charleroi, she was asked to run a Red Cross hospital staffed by volunteer nurses. After being captured by the Germans and transported to Denmark, Violetta made her way to Russia, via Sweden and Finland, where she offered her services to the Russian Red Cross. She worked as part of a "flying column," or mobile army medical unit, facing great danger and hardship in the course of her work. In one section of her memoir, she describes how the flying column arrived at a new temporary base:

"As we neared Radzivilow the guns were crashing away as they did at Lodz, and we prepared for a hot time. The station had been entirely wrecked and was simply in ruins, but the stationmaster's house nearby was still intact, and we had orders to rig up a temporary dressing-station there. Before we had time to unpack our dressings, a messenger arrived to tell us that the Germans had succeeded in enfilading a Russian trench close by, and that they were bringing fifty very badly wounded men to us almost at once. We had just time to start the sterilizer when the little carts began to arrive with some terribly wounded men. The machine guns had simply swept the trench from end to end. The worst of it was that some lived for hours when death would have been a merciful release. Thank God we had plenty of morphia with us and could thus ease their terrible sufferings. One man had practically his whole face blown off, another had all his clothes and the flesh of his back all torn away."

"The shells were crashing over our heads and bursting everywhere, but we were too busy to heed them, as more and more men were brought to the dressing-station."

Violetta Thurstan

Extract from Field Hospital and Flying Column: Being the Journal of an English Nursing Sister in Belgium and Russia *(1915)*

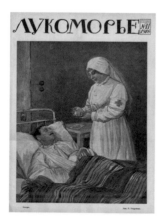
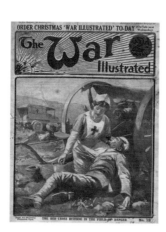
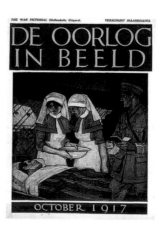
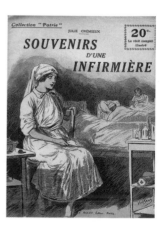

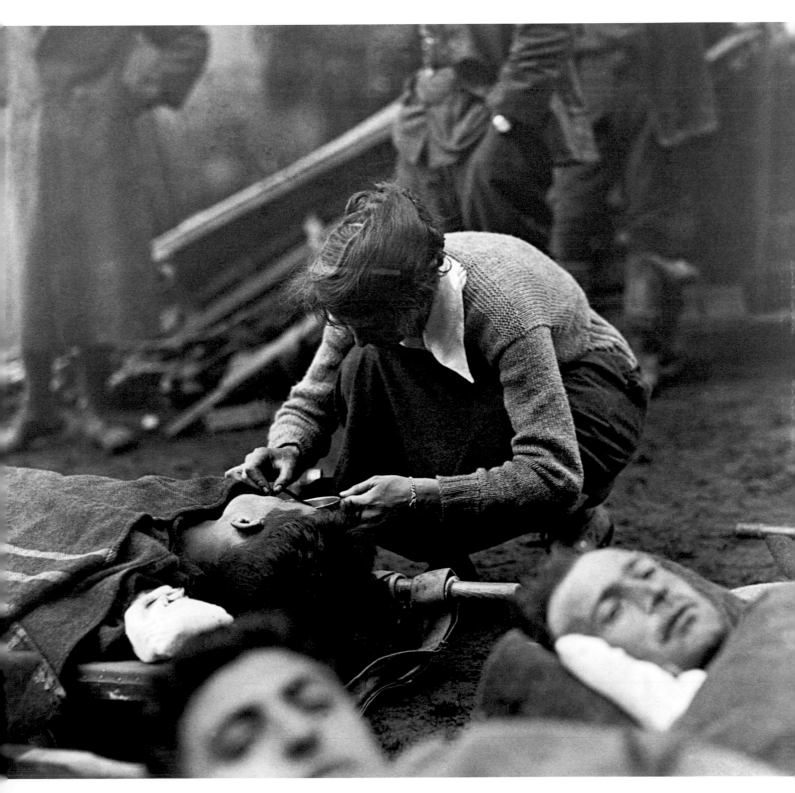

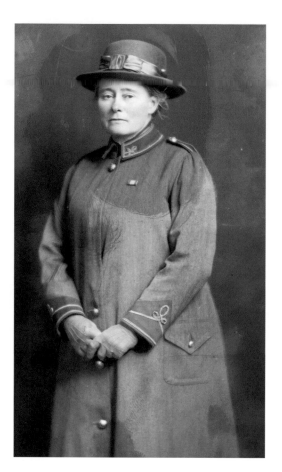

Right:

*Hester Maclean was
Matron-in-Chief of the
New Zealand Army
Nursing Service during
the First World War.*

Opposite:

The Execution of Edith
Cavell *(1865-1915),
engraving from* Le Petit
Journal, *November 1915.
British nurse Edith Cavell
was shot as a spy on
October 12, 1915, because
of her participation in an
underground network that
helped British, French, and
Belgian soldiers to escape
capture. Her famous words,
spoken just before her
execution, have made her an
iconic symbol of pacifism.*

Hester Maclean (1859–1932)

Australian-born Hester Maclean was highly influential in the New Zealand nursing profession. She was Matron of the Queen Victoria Hospital for Women and Children in the Australian province of Victoria. In 1906, she was offered the post of Deputy Inspector of Hospitals and Deputy Registrar of Nurses and Midwives in New Zealand. Hester did some remarkable work as Matron-in-Chief of the New Zealand Army Nursing Services during the First World War, traveling in person with the first contingent of nurses to leave New Zealand for Egypt in 1915. Her whole life was devoted to the development of the nursing profession in New Zealand. Not only was she Deputy Registrar of Nurses, and Matron-in-Chief of the Army Nursing Service, she was also the founder and editor of New Zealand nurses' first dedicated journal, *Kai Tiaki* (see page 89).

Edith Cavell (1865–1915)

The British nurse Edith Cavell is famous because of the way she died—shot as a spy, at dawn on October 12, 1915. She had been a prominent member of an underground network in Brussels that had helped British, Belgian, and French soldiers to escape capture by the Germans in the early months of the First World War. Edith, along with about seventy others who had been part of the underground network, was captured by the Germans, but only Edith and one other were shot. Edith's death was an enormous propaganda coup for the Allies, and it is quite likely that the horror aroused by this incident was one of the things that helped persuade the USA to enter the war in April 1917.

It is, in many ways, a pity that Edith is remembered for her death rather than for her life because she did some remarkable work. The daughter of a vicar, she spent her childhood in the peaceful countryside around her home in Swardeston in the English county of Norfolk. She was educated by governesses, and then, from the age of sixteen, at boarding schools in London, Bristol, and Peterborough. Edith excelled at French, and, after having worked for some years as governess to families in Britain, she took, in 1890, the post of governess to the children of a prominent lawyer in Brussels.

In 1895, Edith decided to become a nurse. She worked first at the Fountain Fever Hospital in South London, England, but soon realized that, if she was to make her way in what was a rapidly developing profession, she would need to obtain formal training. In April 1896, she applied to the training school run by Matron Eva Luckes at the London Hospital in Whitechapel. Edith's early years as a nurse were difficult. Due to her financial circumstances, she had not been able to train as a "special probationer." In many ways, this was a good thing, as she gained a great deal from the two-year training program followed by two years working on the hospital staff and as a private-duty nurse. However, it also meant that she did not automatically gain a prestigious post after qualification, but instead moved from one poorly resourced

infirmary to another. Eventually, Edith's lucky
break came when the family she had worked for
years before, recommended her for work with
leading Brussels surgeon, Antoine Depage. She
was soon invited to lead a new school of nursing,
through which she was to develop nurse training
along the lines of that offered at the London
Hospital. Her school, on the Rue de la Culture,
came to be known as the Berkendael Institute.
Edith ran the Berkendael from 1907 until her capture by the Germans in 1915.

Edith Cavell is believed to have condemned herself by the totally honest responses she gave to
her German interrogators during her imprisonment. Just before her execution she is believed
to have said:

*"But this I would say,
standing before God
and Eternity: I realize
that patriotism is not
enough—I must have
no hatred or bitterness
toward anyone."*

Edith Cavell

Words spoken before her execution (1915)

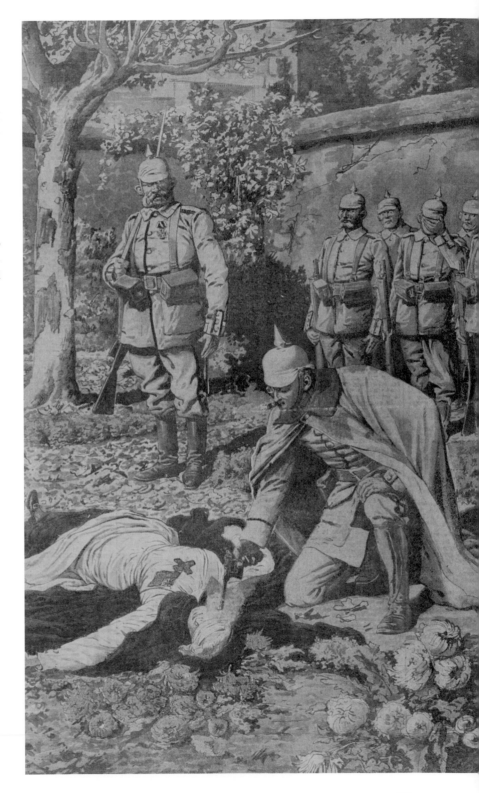

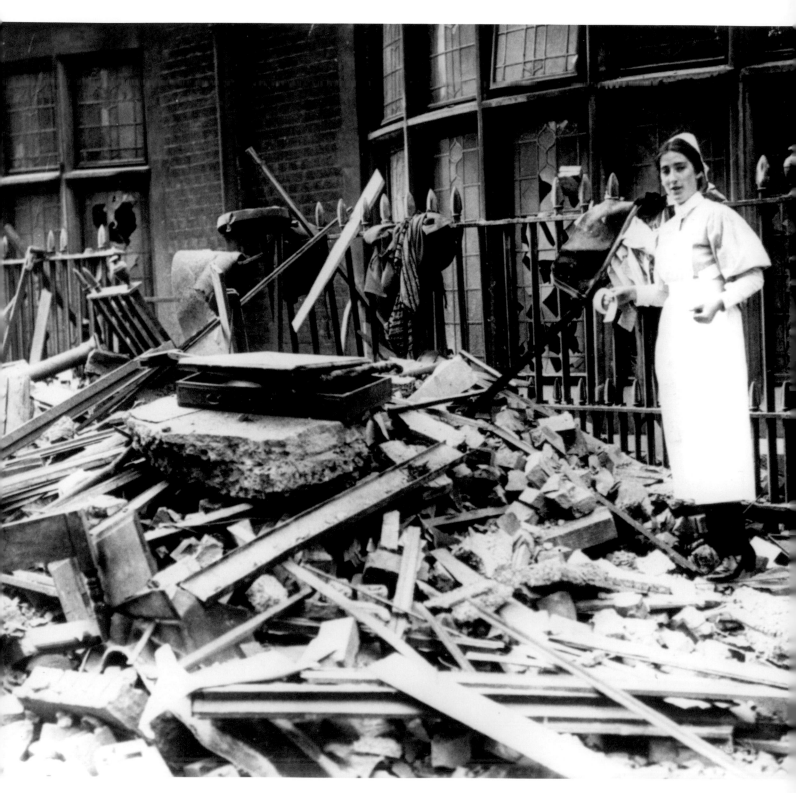

SECOND WORLD WAR (1939–1945)

If the "Great War" had been the first industrial war, then the Second World War went one step further, letting loose its destruction on civilian populations. In 1940, the distinction between front line and home front broke down, as nurses cared for civilian victims of enemy attacks during the "Blitz" and were at risk themselves when hospitals in large cities were relentlessly bombed. In the British city of Coventry, intensive bombing created firestorms that completely destroyed large sections of the city. Three individuals at the Coventry and Warwickshire Hospital—the

Matron, one sister, and the hospital House Governor—were awarded the George Medal for gallantry, but it was said that they were merely representative of the staff as a whole, all of whom acted with great courage and calmness as their hospital was bombed and the nursing home razed to the ground. In British cities, district nurses continued their rounds. Those working at night were at great risk. During the blackouts they were allowed to let only a tiny amount of light from their bicycle lamps guide them as they negotiated their way around the rubble and huge craters created by the falling bombs.

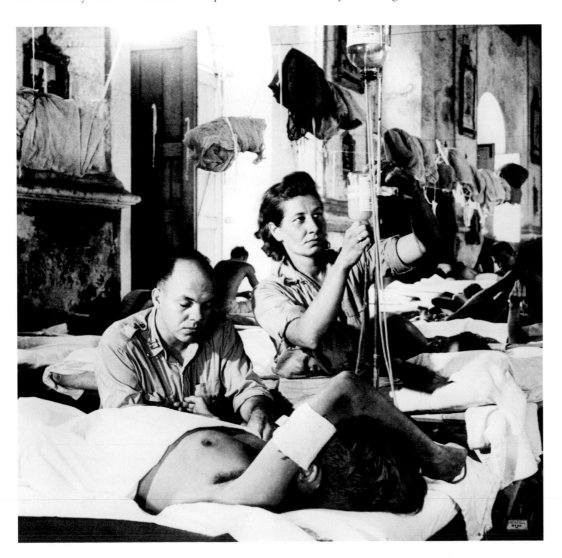

Opposite:
A nurse surveys the damage caused by the blitz in London.

Left:
In December 1944, Leyte Cathedral in the Philippines was converted into an evacuation hospital. Here, army nurse Captain Catherine Acorn, and doctor, Captain D.E. Campbell, attend a wounded man.

Northern France

In the disastrous spring of 1940, nurses in Northern France retreated alongside troops to Dunkirk, many only narrowly escaping capture as their ambulances lurched along bomb-cratered roads. Once back in Britain, they cared for the wounded in their thousands in hastily converted civilian hospitals, as well as in specialist British military hospitals such as Netley Hospital on Southampton Water, and the Royal Herbert Hospital in Woolwich. Nurses worked on hospital ships in the Mediterranean, many losing their lives when their vessels were torpedoed. When the *Strathallan* was struck by a torpedo off Algiers, in November 1942, Olive Stewardson and Julie Kerr, both sisters with the British Queen Alexandra's Imperial Military Nursing Service, immediately went below decks to care for helpless stretcher cases and engine room crew with severe burns. Fortunately, the ship sank very slowly, which meant that it was possible to get all of their patients to safety. The two nurses were awarded the Royal Red Cross in recognition of their bravery.

North Africa, Greece, and Malta

In North Africa, nurses cared for the wounded in Tobruk, while German aircraft dropped bombs on the city. After the Allied victory at El Alamein, Egypt, they joined the advance, receiving the battle wounded in tented casualty clearing stations as close as possible to the front line. Here they cared for badly wounded foot-soldiers, tank personnel with gruesome burns and mutilating injuries, and German prisoners-of-war. In Greece, nurses had to abandon their posts and run for the safety of departing ships as the Italian forces swept through the country, and in Malta nurses took refuge with civilians in caves and tunnels as the island was bombed and strafed by enemy aircraft.

In 1943, penicillin was introduced into military hospitals. It seemed a miracle cure for the dreadfully infected, often gangrenous, wounds that nurses saw in their thousands. Applied to such wounds as a musty-smelling yellow powder, its effects were rapid. It could also be given in injection form, and was used in this way to cure a severe bout of pneumonia contracted by British Prime Minister Winston Churchill.

The Far East

Nurses working in Singapore had a particularly difficult time. When the city fell in 1942, many escaped by sea, but were subsequently shipwrecked when their vessels were attacked by enemy planes, torpedoed, or struck by mines. Many were lost at sea. Others survived on life rafts, to reach islands in the Java Sea, or the mainland of Sumatra, but were subsequently captured by the Japanese and interned in prisoner-of-war camps until the end of the war. It is to the great credit of these trained nurses that they continued

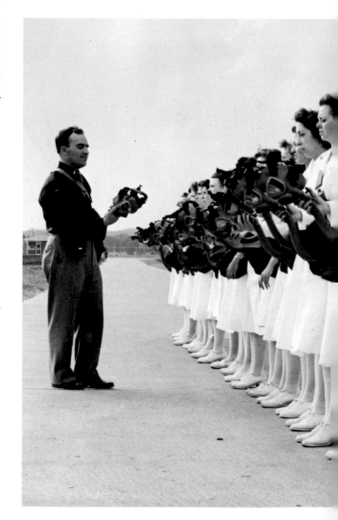

their work in the camps, doing everything they could to help civilians who were desperately sick with life-threatening diseases such as dysentery, typhoid, and malaria. There was little they could do without medicines or equipment, but they worked hard to sustain both the physical health and the morale of their fellow-prisoners. Desperately weak, often ill, and suffering themselves from diseases of malnutrition such as beri-beri, they continued their work for as long as they were physically able, though many died in the process.

D-Day Landings
Nurses were part of the D-Day landings on the French coast of Normandy in June 1944. They staffed hospital ships that navigated the English Channel just behind the troop ships and moved in close to the beaches to receive the wounded. As troops pushed their way inland, medical contingents followed them, setting up casualty clearing stations en route to the Rhine. Some of the most seriously wounded were returned to Britain via Dakota aircraft. Nurses who volunteered for duty as flying nurse attendants had a challenging job. They accompanied severely injured patients during the long journey home across the English Channel, changing their dressings, controlling their bleeding, and replacing lost fluids through intravenous drips. Their meticulous attention to detail doubtless saved many lives.

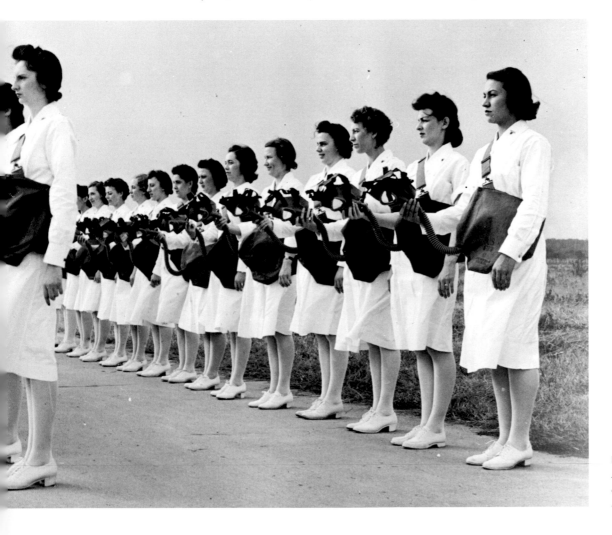

Left:
*American nurses undergoing
a gas mask drill during the
Second World War.*

Brenda McBryde

British nurse Brenda McBryde wrote a compelling memoir of her years with Britain's Queen Alexandra's Imperial Military Nursing Service during the Second World War. In her writing, she managed to capture the skill and artistry of nursing work. On one occasion she and a colleague cared for a ward full of newly arrived wounded men in a tented hospital in France. She wrote of a corporal who was:

"half comatosed, with an uncertain grip on life... Gently, we eased him out of his jacket and what was left of his trousers, still caked in mud from the hole where he had lain, and we rolled him on to his good side. There is not much room to manoeuvre on a stretcher and I cradled him firmly to me while Joan soaped and gently sponged his back, all reddened and pitted with bits of earth and grass."

With great care, the nurses washed the patient and put him into clean pajamas. They then pinned sterile towels onto the front of their dresses and dressed his wounds using an aseptic technique to avoid introducing any new infection. After cleaning his mouth and combing his hair, they ended by giving the patient an injection of penicillin and leaving him to sleep before moving to the next wounded man. The whole process had taken forty minutes and there was a ward full of patients waiting for them.

The nurses fed the unconscious and severely traumatized patients through nasogastric tubes that ran through the nose and directly into the stomach. Through these tubes they carefully poured egg, milk, glucose, and casein. Unconscious patients were catheterized, and nurses kept a careful record of how much urine they produced, to make sure they were giving enough fluids to avoid dehydration. Every two hours, patients were turned from side to side to avoid pressure sores. Their mouths were cleaned regularly and gauze masks were placed over their faces to protect them from flies. Once the patients were awake, their tubes could be removed, and they could be carefully spoon-fed until they were well enough to feed themselves.

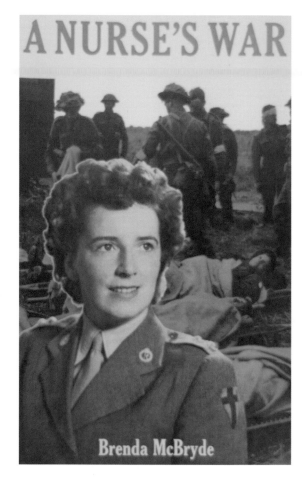

A NURSE'S WAR

Brenda McBryde

This care was amazingly labour-intensive, and nurses worked long shifts in order to get through the work.

After the end of the war, Brenda worked in a hospital in Celle, Germany, which had just taken in starving and emaciated patients from a nearby concentration camp. She described the effort of trying to "connect" emotionally with people who had lost all trust for their fellow human beings. Although many were seriously ill with conditions such as heart failure, bronchitis, and liver abscesses, nurses did not insist that they stay in bed, but allowed them as much freedom as they felt they needed. In addition to dressing wounds and giving medications, the nurses handed out vitamin tablets and weaned their malnourished patients onto a full diet.

Right:

The front cover of Brenda McBryde's evocative book, which recounts her experiences as an army nurse during the Second World War. The book is not just an account of nursing work in all its intricacies. It is also a compelling record of the Second World War, seen through the eyes of someone who witnessed its true horrors.

Opposite:

An Australian field tent hospital.

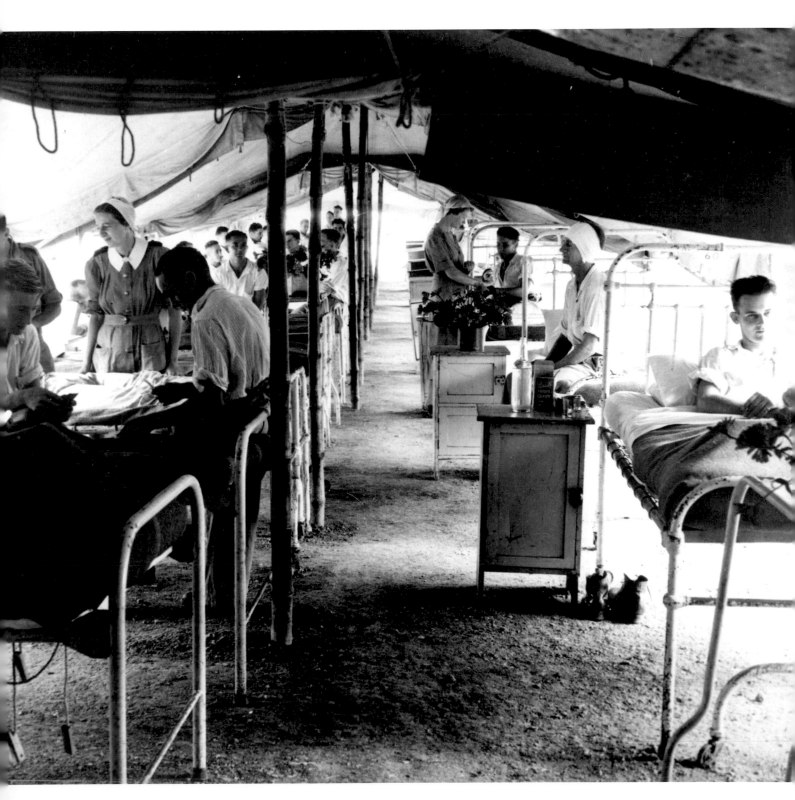

KOREAN WAR (1950–1953)

The Korean War, ostensibly fought between North and South Korea, was really one highly combative element of the "Cold War" between Russia and the West. When the Russian-supported Communist state of North Korea moved across the 28th parallel and invaded the South, the United Nations mobilized a force composed of troops from twenty-two nations. British nurses served on board the hospital ship *Maine II*, which took injured combatants from the port of Pusan to Japan. Most of the patients were American GIs with terrible injuries. Many had severe gangrene, acquired on the Korean fields, which were manured with human excrement.

When conditions allowed, amputations were done on board ship, and severely traumatized patients were kept alive by the constant attentions of nurses until they reached the safety of a hospital. These nurses also cared for victims of napalm

bombs (many of them injured by "wrongly aimed" air attacks). Always severely burned, these patients required intensive nursing care if they were to survive.

American military nurses were developing techniques for the care and treatment of patients with life-threatening injuries. In the fall of 1950, three superbly equipped American hospital ships, the *Repose, Haven,* and *Consolation* arrived at Pusan, allowing the hard-pressed *Maine II* to take a large contingent of severely burned patients to Hong Kong.

The Korean War was a terrible conflict in which numerous atrocities were committed against civilians. Nurses had to be capable of caring for patients suffering not only from physical injury but also from a form of "battle fatigue" that was brought on by the mental suffering of troops who were all too aware of the brutality and futility of the war.

Right:
An army nurse cares for a wounded soldier in Korea, c. 1953.

Opposite:
Mary Ann Krisman-Scott worked as a US Army nurse during the Vietnam War. She cared for patients with severe physical wounds, many of whom also suffered from post-traumatic stress disorder.

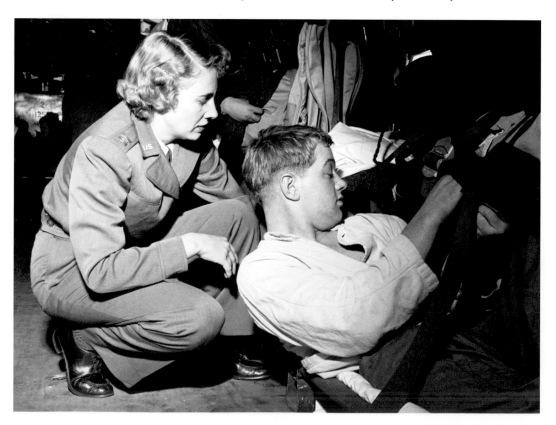

VIETNAM WAR (1959–1973)

American nurses were first assigned to Vietnam in the early 1960s. Due to the rapidly rising casualty rate, their numbers were increased in 1966, in spite of recruitment difficulties caused by the unpopularity of the war. The Navy Nurse Corps played a significant role in caring for the wounded. Two veteran hospital ships, the *Repose* and the *Sanctuary,* provided important care to severely wounded troops, carrying highly trained personnel and the most up-to-date medical equipment.

In September 1966 a bill was passed authorizing the recruitment of male nurses to the regular Army, Navy, and Air Force Nurse Corps, and large numbers of male nurses were subsequently recruited. Many of them worked in theaters, some as anesthetists; others specialized in psychiatry.

Semipermanent hospitals were built housing the latest technology, yet ready to evacuate at any moment. Patients were transported to these hospitals very rapidly, via helicopter, and survival rates surpassed those of any previous war. After the signing of the ceasefire in January 1973, nurses in Veterans Administration hospitals did important work in enabling former combatants to overcome the debilitating mental illnesses associated with combat in what had been seen as such a futile war. Many became expert in the care of patients with post-traumatic stress disorder.

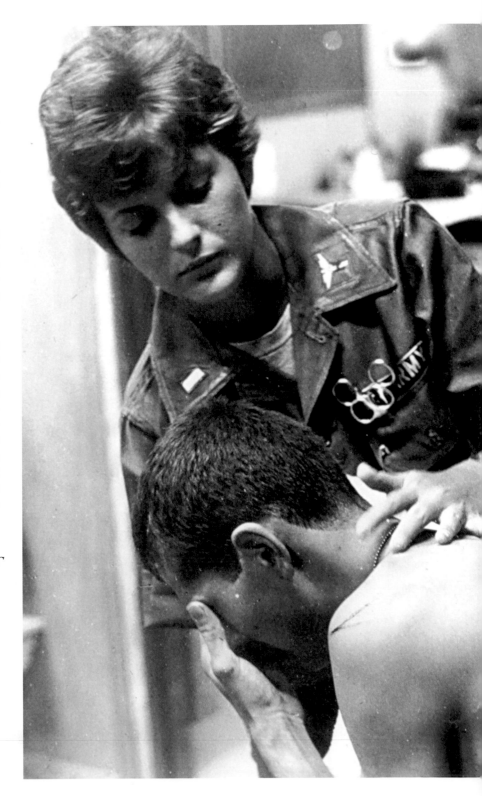

> *"Sometimes the wounds of war are not visible, but they remain just as painful. Nurses always care for both."*

Mary Ann Krisman-Scott

Former US Military Nurse

DISASTER AND CONFLICT IN THE MODERN AGE

The First Iraq War offered nurses a testing environment in which to practice their skills. Iraq invaded Kuwait on August 2, 1990, and when it refused to leave, a US-led coalition, acting on behalf of the United Nations, mounted Operation Desert Storm, in which Iraqi forces were driven out of Kuwait.

Nurses were deployed throughout the area of operations, often close to the front lines. They set up tented MASH (Mobile Army Surgical Hospital) units, and cared for injured civilians as well as troops. Their work required a high level of initiative and a capacity for improvisation. Nurses were involved in triage (assessing patients as they arrived at the unit, and deciding who needed the most urgent treatment). They also prepared patients for—and assisted in—complex surgery, and operated state-of-the-art life-support equipment.

In the last decades of the twentieth century, nurses were to be found wherever there was a war, a terrorist attack, or any other form of humanitarian crisis. Traveling as part of army nursing corps, and with charitable and humanitarian organizations such as Médecins Sans Frontières and the International Red Cross, nurses offered core nursing care and high-tech medical treatments. Their rapid intervention saved many lives.

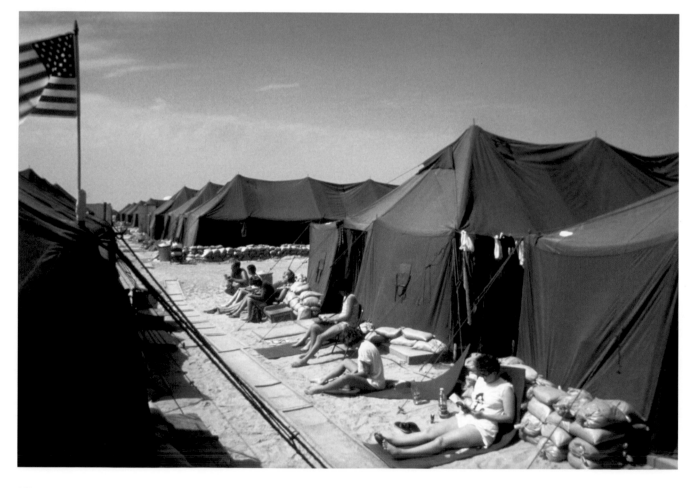

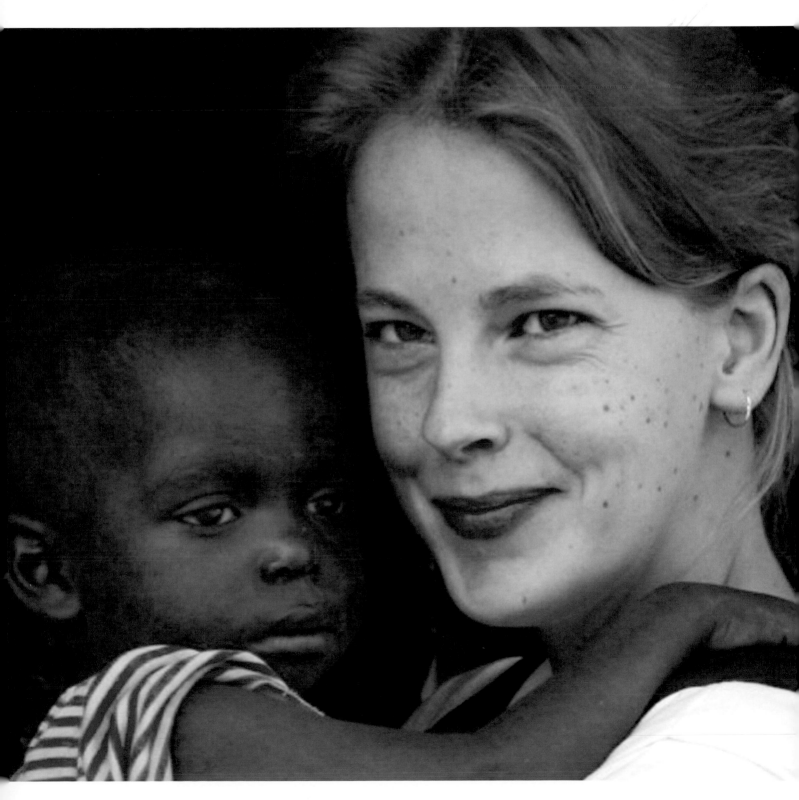

As Seen On Screen

Ever since the mass media of film and then television became popular in the twentieth century, stereotypical images of nurses have been portrayed. Most frequently nurses have been depicted as "angel," "heroine," "mother," or "whore." Even before the invention of film, extreme images of nurses were portrayed in poetry and fiction. On the one hand, there were the nineteenth-century "unreformed" nurses epitomized by Sairey Gamp in the English writer Charles Dickens's novel *Martin Chuzzlewit*. Such fictional pen-portraits were, ostensibly, an attempt to promote the reform of nursing in the mid-nineteenth century. Yet Dickens's portrayal of gin-swilling, self-centered, and uncaring nurses did a disservice to the many well-intentioned and hardworking nurses of his day. At the other end of the scale, Florence Nightingale found herself the subject of poems praising her "saintly" qualities. Notable among these was "Santa Filomena," by the American poet Henry Wadsworth Longfellow.

NURSES ON FILM

The first two decades of the twentieth century saw the advent of silent films, containing portrayals of the "romantic nurse," in which the love interest rather than the nursing was emphasized. Many were melodramas based around the aftermath of the First World War in which wounded heroes were nursed by emotional females.

Nursing as First World War Propaganda

The work carried out by nurses who served in the war did much to create the image of the nurse as pure yet immensely courageous and powerful. The nurse was now a fully fledged "angel of mercy," who could brave the battlefield to save lives and heal wounds. In their writings on the portrayal of nurses in popular culture, American authors Philip and Beatrice Kalisch have argued that:

"World War I saw the last glorious outpouring of the angel of mercy imagery that had persisted since the time of Nightingale."

The greatest Allied propaganda coup of the war was the portrayal of the execution of the British Nurse Edith Cavell in films such as *Nurse and Martyr* and *The Martyrdom of Nurse Cavell*. As these titles imply, Edith was more than just a saint—she had actually died for the Allied cause. It is quite possible that Edith herself would have been shocked at the way in which her story was distorted for propaganda purposes. This image of her was overturned when a statue was erected to her in London. Initially inscribed *For King and Country*, it eventually came to bear Edith's own words (see page 133).

The Interwar Years

The heroic image of nurses in film persisted after the war. In the 1930s the nurse was portrayed as a serious professional woman with an important job to do. As Lora in *Night Nurse* (1931), Barbara Stanwyck was a true heroine, rescuing her patients from a criminal doctor. One of the most remarkable American films of this time, however, was *The Storm* (1930), in which a nurse performs emergency surgery on board a ship lost in a storm at sea.

The Second World War Nurse

In the early 1940s, war once again brought the heroic nurse to the fore. In both Britain and the USA, nurses were portrayed as an asset to the war effort—patriotic, brave, and hardworking. The American film, *To the Shores of Tripoli* (1942), portrays a competent Navy nurse, played by Maureen O'Hara, who is keenly aware of her officer status and has a strong sense of duty and integrity. One of the most dramatic films of the war, *So Proudly We Hail* (1943), depicts the harrowing experiences of American nurses in Corregidor (in the Philippines), one of whom sacrifices her own life to save the others.

The Nurse in Postwar Films

The nurse in postwar films was a domestic icon: a mother-figure. Men still fell in love with her, but now they saw her as a symbol of security, a "safe haven." In *The Hasty Heart* (1950) a nurse becomes emotionally involved with a dying patient, yet manages to keep a safe, professional distance. In such films, nurses act as the catalysts who allow men to find salvation: nurses restore confidence in life and humanity.

In Britain, the 1950s saw a remarkable celebration of iconic saintly nurses, with a depiction by the famous actress Anna Neagle of Florence Nightingale in the film *The Lady with a Lamp* (1951) (Neagle had also portrayed Edith Cavell in the 1939 film, *Nurse Edith Cavell*). These strong, if rather sanitized, portrayals were popular with audiences, who wanted to see their nurses as admirable human beings. The British film, *The Feminine Touch* (1958), follows a group of nurse-trainees. Rather predictably, the heroine, Susan, marries a doctor and leaves nursing. Yet the film portrays nurses as strong—if rather "sweet"—humane, and full of character.

Below:
A still from the 1939 film Nurse Edith Cavell, *starring British actress Anna Neagle.*

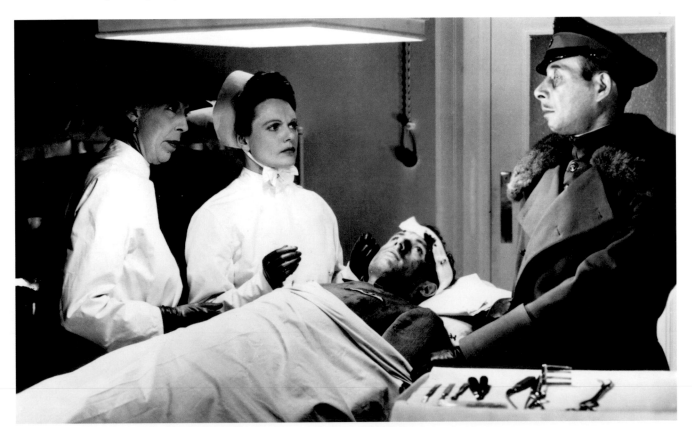

The "Naughty Nurse"

The mid-century portrayal of nurses as objects of romantic interest shifted in the new atmosphere of the 1960s. In an era of sexual liberation, nurses became objects of media exploitation. Perhaps because of their handling of patients' bodies and the apparent intimacy this created, nurses were portrayed as highly sexualized by a media industry that was going through its own peculiar kind of adolescence.

The British "Carry On" series of films, although lampooning many professionals and public stereotypes of its day, found nurses a particularly easy target for comedy. In *Carry On Nurse* (1959) there is a sense that nurses are still competent and confident mother figures, yet there is also a shift to a more risqué portrayal than before. In the later film, *Carry On Matron* (1972), the nurse is depicted as highly sexualized and flirtatious. Beginning as innocent comedies, the "Carry On" films rapidly became highly farcical and quite destructive to the images of those they were "exposing." The most memorable nurse figures in these films are Nurse Sandra May, played by Barbara Windsor, and Matron, played by Hattie Jacques. Both are portrayed as "sex-mad" and highly unprofessional figures.

Opposite:

Filming an episode of the American television series, MASH.

Below:

Publicity poster for The Lady with a Lamp *(1951), featuring British actress Anna Neagle as Florence Nightingale.*

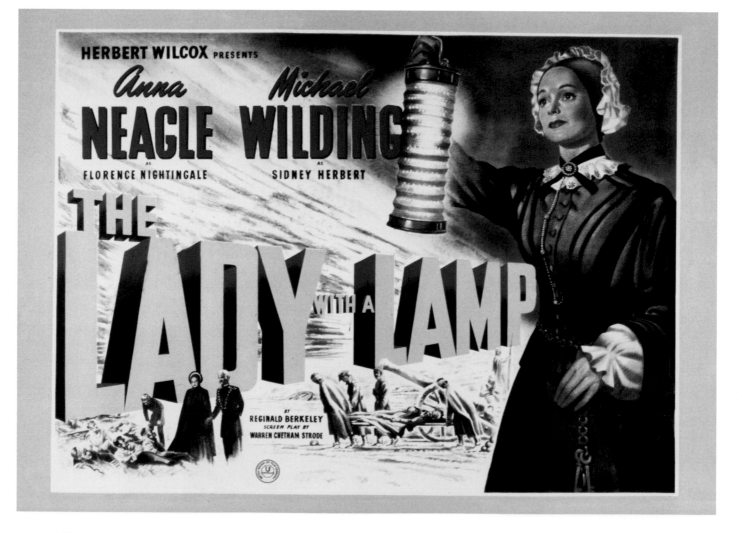

The Demonic Nurse

In the 1970 American film, *MASH*, set in the 1950s during the Korean War, nurses are portrayed as sexually predatory and emotionally closed. Major Margaret "Hotlips" Houlihan, a hypocritical disciplinarian, gets her come-uppance when the "heroes" of the film, Hawkeye and Duke, play a practical joke on her. Nurses in 1970s films and TV series were often frightening figures whose power over the intimate bodily functions of their vulnerable patients was seen, for the first time, as a threat. Nurses were no longer heroically or angelically powerful. They were now "demonically" so.

Frightening films such as *The Honeymoon Killers* (1970), *One Flew Over the Cuckoo's Nest* (1975), and *Misery* (1990) portray nurses as sadists and monsters. Patients are defenseless, though they do attempt to rebel against the nurse's cruelty. With their highly inaccurate portrayals of nurses, these films tapped into the fears of a generation of viewers and damaged the professional reputations of real-life nurses. In some ways, though, they illustrated, even more than the angelic portrayals of the early twentieth century, how powerful people believed nurses to be. They asked the question: What would life be like if nurses were *not* altruistic human beings with high professional standards?

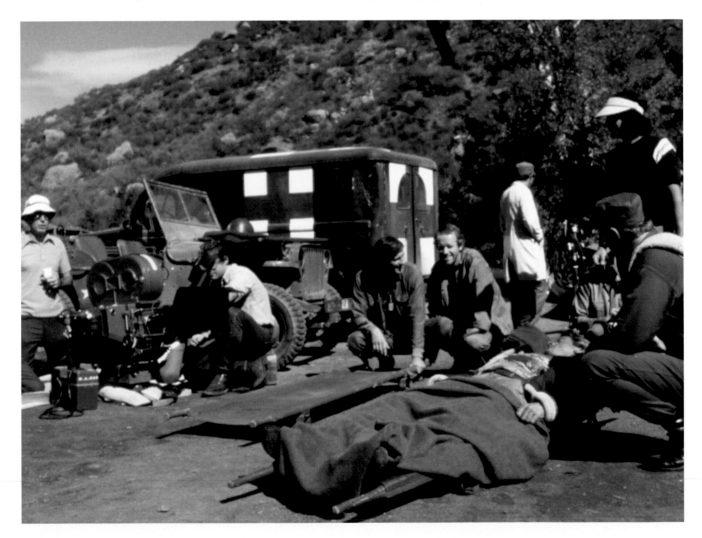

NURSES ON TV

The 1960s saw the rise of the medical drama, epitomized by the immensely popular long-running American television series, *Dr Kildare*. As in other TV serials of its time, *Dr Kildare* portrayed brilliant creative doctors and pretty but nondescript nurses, who merely followed the doctors' orders, while at the same time falling in love with them. In this way, television dramas from the mid century depicted nurses as little more than doctors' assistants and the objects of romance.

The Professional Nurse

It was only during the 1980s and 1990s that these stereotypical images of nurses were discredited. The Second Wave feminist movement of the 1970s had campaigned against negative portrayals of women. Even more importantly, it was becoming clear to policy-makers that the prevailing media portrayal of nurses could threaten the profession (and everyone's health) by making nursing unattractive to well-educated and thoughtful young people. A social backlash against the gross misrepresentation of nurses followed.

This trend began as early as the 1970s. Television dramas such as *Angels* in Britain attempted to offer realistic portrayals of nurses struggling to reconcile their public images and private lives. The historical drama, *District Nurse*, presented the nurse as a wise but deferential altruist at the heart of her community. The long-running British television soap opera *Casualty* was often deliberately political, emphasizing the poor pay and conditions of nurses, yet it rarely demeaned or devalued nurses, showing them instead as the lynchpin of the Accident and Emergency Department. The head nurse, Charlie Fairhead, was presented as an iconic nurse for the twentieth century. And in the USA, the character of the nurse-practitioner, Carol Hathaway, depicted by Julianna Margulies in *ER,* demonstrated the adoption of more serious and independent roles by nurses toward the end of the century.

In recent years British TV producers have become interested in nursing's past. *Casualty 1907, Casualty 1908,* and *Casualty 1909* portrayed life and work at the London Hospital in the early twentieth century. The popularity of this new departure into historical "docu-drama" illustrates a sense of longing for a bygone era. Such nostalgia is typical of societies who all too often fail to reward the nurses of their own time.

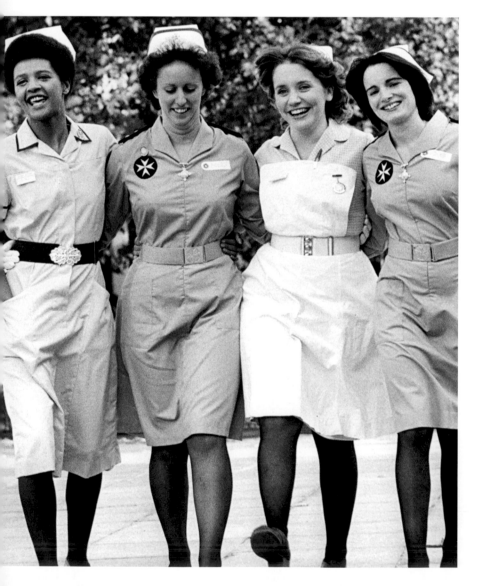

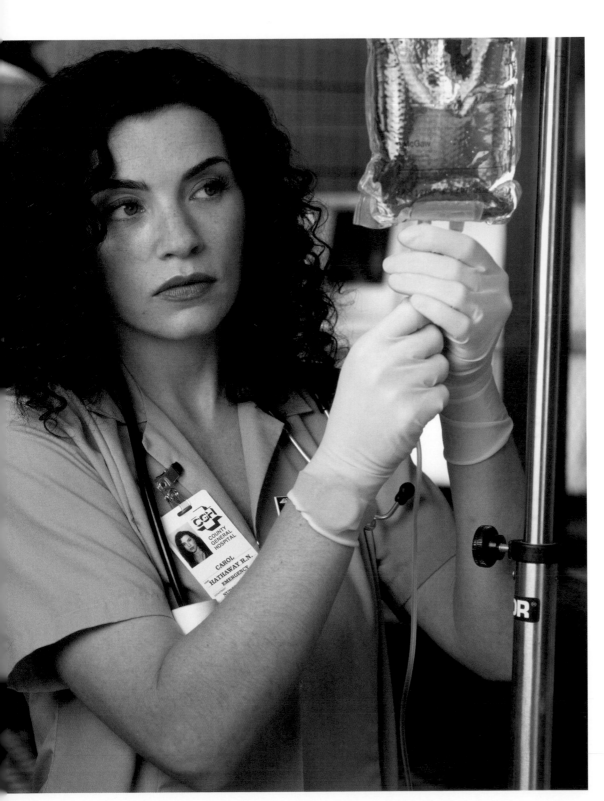

Left:
*Julianna Margulies as
Nurse Carol Hathaway in
the popular US television
series, ER.*

Opposite:
*Photograph taken during
a St John Ambulance (SJA)
celebration of nursing.
In the image are (left to
right): Angela Bruce (actress
in the British BBC TV
series, Angels); Mrs. S.
Jackson (State Registered
Nurse); Joanna Monro
(also from Angels); and
Lyn Domniguez (St John
Ambulance volunteer).
The white Maltese crosses
on the SJA uniforms date
back to the Knights
Hospitallers of St John of
Jerusalem (see pages
20–21).*

New Technology and New Roles

The twentieth century saw dramatic changes in the work of nurses. As new technology was invented, nurses found ways of making it useful for patients. Among the most significant changes were those that involved monitoring patients' conditions. At the turn of the century, nurses were able to measure pulse, blood pressure, and temperature. Using these techniques, they could assess whether a patient might have an infection or be at risk of collapse. By the end of the century, much more nuanced diagnostic equipment was available. Nurses were now using more efficient sphygmomanometers (measuring blood pressure) and were routinely reading electrocardiograms (measuring heart function). In intensive care units, they were monitoring their patients' changing status through a range of respiratory and heart monitors, as well as taking frequent blood tests and measuring patients' fluid intake and output.

ROLE EXPANSION

As the century progressed, nurses took on increasing responsibility for monitoring their patients' conditions. They reported their findings to doctors, but also assessed for themselves the changes that were taking place inside their patients' bodies, and were ready to act rapidly on their assessments.

The two world wars had a significant impact on the development of health technologies. During the First World War, the process of blood transfusion, invented decades earlier, was developed by Canadian military doctors. By the end of the war, quite large numbers of "collapsed" patients were receiving transfusions. During the Second World War, nurses became responsible for administering this treatment and for monitoring patients for signs of "rejection" or "shock."

In the USA, nurse-anesthetists were beginning to practice just prior to the First World War. They brought their knowledge and skills to the hospitals of the Western Front when America entered the war in April 1917. Around this time, British, Australian, New Zealand, and South African nurses were also being trained as anesthetists. They practiced in casualty clearing stations close to the front lines, and their work helped save many lives. To their disappointment, all but the American nurses had this role removed from them after the war (Australians were not allowed to practice as anesthetists, even during the conflict). Anesthesiology became a jealously protected medical role once more, even though nurses had proved that they were competent to do the work.

THE IRON LUNG

The earliest clinically effective iron lung, or negative pressure ventilator, was developed in the 1920s by the Americans Philip Drinker and Charles McKhann. The machine was used to keep alive patients whose breathing muscles—in the chest wall and diaphragm—were paralyzed. The patient was placed in a large cylindrical steel container, with only the head and neck free at one end. The air pressure inside the cylinder was alternately raised and lowered so that the chest wall was drawn outward and then pushed back down. This caused air to be drawn into and then pushed out of the lungs. The greatest use for the iron lung came

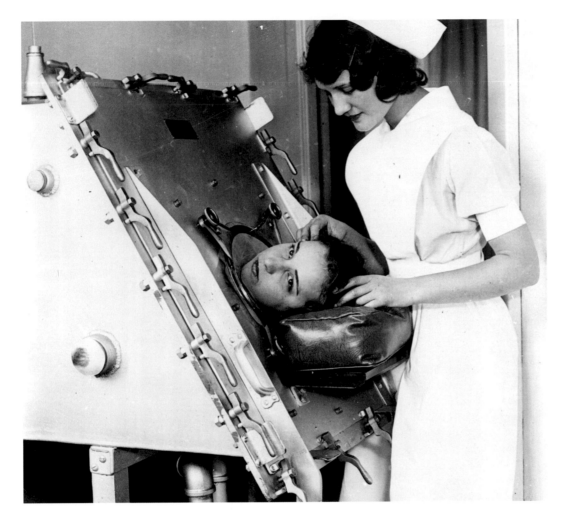

Student nurses Ruth Hillier and Donna Brewer, of the San Francisco Children's Hospital, demonstrate the use of the "Drinker Respirator" in the late 1920s. The apparatus was used to keep patients alive for weeks after normal respiration had ceased.

mid-century, when there were frequent epidemics of poliomyelitis (or "polio"), during which breathing muscles could become paralyzed, causing patients to die of suffocation.

The iron lung was first used for a child with respiratory failure at the Boston Children's Hospital in 1928. A less expensive model was invented by John Emerson in 1931, and during the polio epidemics of the mid-twentieth century, whole wards could be filled with the new style of ventilator. Patients were kept on the iron lung until their bodies were able to fight off the polio virus and recover. In the 1950s, the iron lung was superseded by a new form of ventilator that pushed air into the lungs via a tube in the trachea (windpipe). At the same time,

American physicians Jonas Salk and Albert Sabin were developing successful vaccines against polio. Once the vaccine had been developed, polio was almost entirely eradicated from the populations of developed nations.

The use of the iron lung had important implications for nurses. They had to take meticulous care in ensuring that the machine was working correctly and that their patients were receiving the air-supply they needed. They also had to offer important nursing care and emotional reassurance to patients who were effectively trapped in a rigid, sealed cylinder. The need for both technical expertise and sensitivity were paramount, and the care of these patients demanded all of the nurses' skills and abilities.

ANTIBIOTICS

Before the invention of antibiotics, nurses were heavily dependent on antiseptic treatments and aseptic techniques to protect their patients from severe, life-threatening infections. Antisepsis meant the use of potent chemicals that would kill bacteria but might also damage the healthy tissues of the patients on which they were used. Asepsis was a much more effective approach, but could do nothing against an infection that had already taken hold in a patient's body.

Examples of infectious diseases with horrific effects on the world's populations have already been mentioned. One particularly horrible example can be found in the range of wound infections that affected soldiers who were fighting their way across the heavily manured fields of Northern France and Flanders during the First World War. Diseases such as tetanus and gas-gangrene took hold with great rapidity, and many limbs—and lives—were lost. In the interwar period, tuberculosis was widespread, causing thousands of deaths and leaving survivors with permanently damaged lungs.

The Discovery of Penicillin

In 1928, Alexander Fleming, a bacteriologist at St Mary's Hospital, London, was experimenting on certain bacteria when his samples were accidentally contaminated with a mold known as penicillin. To his amazement, he found that the penicillin seemed to kill the bacteria. In this way, he discovered the first effective antibiotic. Other compounds such as streptomycin (effective against tuberculosis) and chloramphenicol (effective against typhoid fever) were rapidly developed.

Although antibiotics were not the first drugs with microbe-killing properties to be discovered (the highly toxic sulphonamides had already been made available), the discovery of antibiotics had a revolutionary effect on the health of entire populations. Quite apart from the fact that many of those who contracted serious infectious diseases lived, when they would previously have died, the availability of antibiotics meant that much more ambitious surgery could now be attempted with safety. Medical and surgical treatment developed rapidly—and with them the role of the nurse, who now prepared patients for, and assisted their recovery from, much more complex treatments.

Nurses were also now dealing with complex, and sometimes life-threatening, side-effects of the antibiotics themselves, and their roles were changing rapidly. First tested on British troops during the North Africa campaign in 1943, penicillin was made available to whole populations in the immediate postwar period. A small minority of patients had a disastrous allergic reaction to the drug that was known as anaphylactic shock, and nurses had to mobilize rapid life-saving responses to this.

"And you see we had to work hard on these things, foot baths, hot fomentations, because we had no antibiotics. And it was nursing…And we had to encourage them to eat and drink… to encourage their appetites, get them to drink water…So antibiotics took over from these kind of treatments for sepsis. It was heavy work but that was how it was."
St Bartholomew's Hospital Nurse (1934)
From The Nurses' Voices Project, University of Kingston-upon-Thames

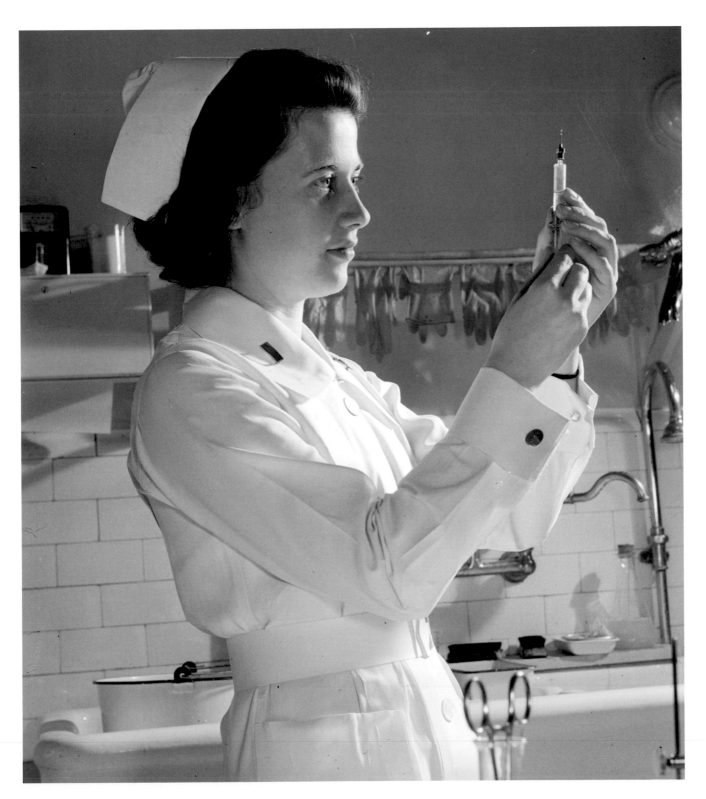

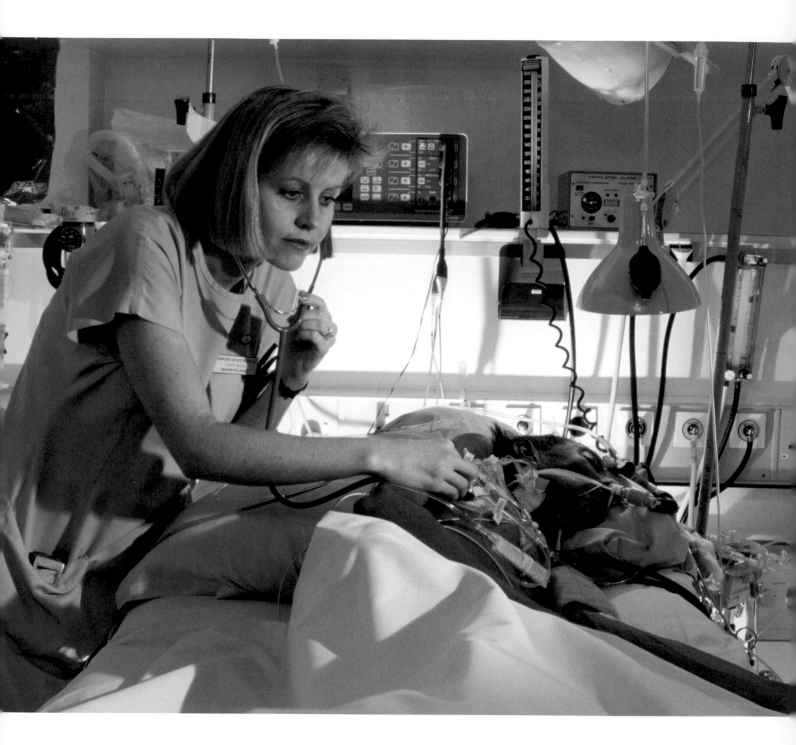

INTENSIVE THERAPY

The introduction into hospitals of machinery for supporting life and monitoring patients' conditions coincided with dramatic changes in the ways in which some nurses worked. However, perhaps surprisingly, intensive care units themselves appeared before sophisticated life-saving machines were invented. US historians Julie Fairman and Joan Lynaugh have shown that the earliest intensive care units were the joint development of nurses and doctors working together at grassroots level on hospital wards. The units began to emerge in the USA during the 1950s, when it became clear that the vigilance—or lack of it—of nurses could determine whether fragile patients lived or died.

A New Type of Hospital Ward

Until just after the Second World War, nurses arranged the patients in their wards so that those who were critically ill were placed in beds closest to the nurse's station, where they could be watched carefully for any signs of deterioration. The rapid advance of private health care came during the mid-century, at a time when privacy (or semiprivacy) was thought desirable; people were willing to pay to be offered health care in a room of their own. Consequently, many hospital wards were restructured with long corridors and separate rooms. This had serious implications for the ability of the nurses to do their job. Patients could have heart attacks or suffer severe hemorrhage out of the nurse's sight behind closed doors. To overcome this problem, nurses and doctors in several hospitals worked closely together, with the help of administrators, to bring critically ill patients into units close to the nurse's station. These were the earliest intensive care units. Importantly, it was often the initiative of nurses that led to their development. Eventually, "intensive care units" and "intensive therapy units" (where slightly more stable patients were cared for) became separate wards, and intensive care nurses were recognized

as specialists. The American Association of Critical Care Nursing was founded in 1969.

Clinical Judgment

Once established, intensive care units became the homes of newly invented complex life-saving machines such as ventilators and monitors. Nurses had to become adept technicians as well as compassionate carers, and the scope of their practice expanded dramatically. They worked very independently in these units, knowing when to act on their own initiative, and when to call a doctor to change a patient's prescribed treatment. Their clinical judgement was pivotal to the patient's survival.

Some of the earliest intensive care units developed out of coronary care units, because it was in coronary care that the most unstable patients were to be found. One of the first units was established by Dr Lawrence Meltzer and nurse Rose Pinneo at the Presbyterian Hospital, Philadelphia, in 1963. They successfully brought together a team of doctors and nurses to work on the unit, teaching and conducting research as well as offering the safest possible care to their patients. In the preface to their textbook, *Intensive Coronary Care*, they pointed out that coronary care was not so much a form of mechanized medicine as a new system of nursing care.

Ethics and Intensive Therapy

Intensive care units and the emergence of critical care undoubtedly saved many lives in the twentieth century. These "advances" also raised ethical and moral issues for nurses and doctors—dilemmas about who to save and who to let die. Many terminally ill patients preferred not to undergo frightening and uncomfortable experiences involving high-tech machinery and resuscitation techniques, and it was in these cases that the artistry of nursing came more to the fore, in assisting pain-free and peaceful death.

Opposite:
A nurse checks on a patient in the intensive care unit of the Princess Grace Hospital in London, England.

SPECIALIST NURSES

Critical care nursing was only one of a number of specialisms that emerged during the course of the twentieth century. In the USA, specialisms developed wherever it became clear that new diseases or new technological advances meant that specialist knowledge and skill was necessary. The earliest group to develop their own systems of examinations and certificates was the American Association of Nurse Anesthetists, which began to issue certificates of competence in 1946. Other groups followed later in the century: the American College of Nurse-Midwives in 1971, the American Association of Critical Care Nurses in 1976, and the National Board of Pediatric Nurse Practitioners and Associates in 1977.

In Britain, the number of nurse-specialist roles increased dramatically in the 1980s and 1990s. During the 1990s, the role of "nurse consultant" began to appear. The British nurse consultant has direct responsibility for a caseload of patients,

advises colleagues, and engages in research and teaching in her or his specialist area.

The Nurse-Practitioner Movement in the USA

During the middle decades of the twentieth century, dramatic changes began to affect the way in which US nurses worked—particularly in community settings and with deprived sections of the population. The introduction of the Medicare and Medicaid systems meant that all citizens were entitled to some form of health care; yet demand threatened to outstrip supply. In order to cope with mushrooming workloads, doctors began to delegate part of their clinical role to nurses. Nurses were, increasingly, undertaking clinical assessments and developing treatment plans for patients with complex chronic diseases.

The change was caused, in part, because nurses in the mid-century were realizing just how much knowledge and skill they possessed. In some areas,

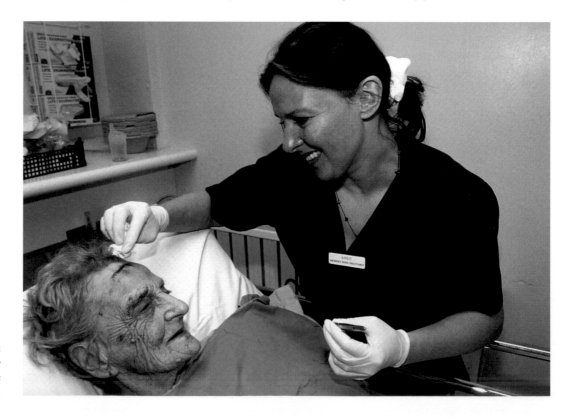

Right:
A British nurse-practitioner tends to an elderly patient's head wound.

their knowledge was equal to that of a junior doctor, while in others (particularly in understanding patients' reactions to illness and treatment) their expertise surpassed that of their doctor-colleagues. They were also, increasingly, asserting that it was part of their role to think creatively and design solutions to their patients' problems rather than simply follow doctors' orders.

The "Doctor–Nurse Game"

In 1967, a psychiatrist called Leonard Stein studied the professional relationships between doctors and nurses. His theory, named "The Doctor–Nurse Game," proposed that experienced nurses were much more knowledgeable and confident than junior doctors, and that nurses would typically "steer" the decision-making of doctors to serve the best interests of their patients. This happened, however, in a very subtle way. So, for example, if an unsure junior doctor seemed to be about to prescribe an ineffective (or even dangerous) treatment, a nurse might ask a question that would

make the doctor reevaluate his or her decision. The problem with this approach was that, although patients often got the treatment they needed, nurses rarely got the credit they deserved. As the century wore on, nurses became impatient with this game and began to offer more direct advice to doctors. This increasing confidence coincided with a rapid increase in the workload of doctors and a tendency for doctors to specialize. Nurses and doctors in many areas—but particularly in general practice—began to feel that it was time to change their practice and to shift their boundaries. Nurses began to work much more independently—especially with chronically ill patients, and in community settings. They undertook complex clinical assessments, diagnosed illness, prescribed treatment, and designed complete plans of care. The advantage of having a nurse to do this kind of work was that she was trained to look at the patient as a whole being, rather than as just a condition or disease, and this enabled her to design a complex "pathway" of care.

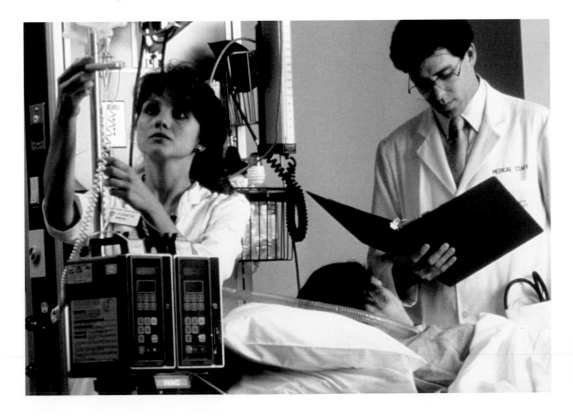

Left:

A doctor and a nurse attend to a patient in a coronary care unit.

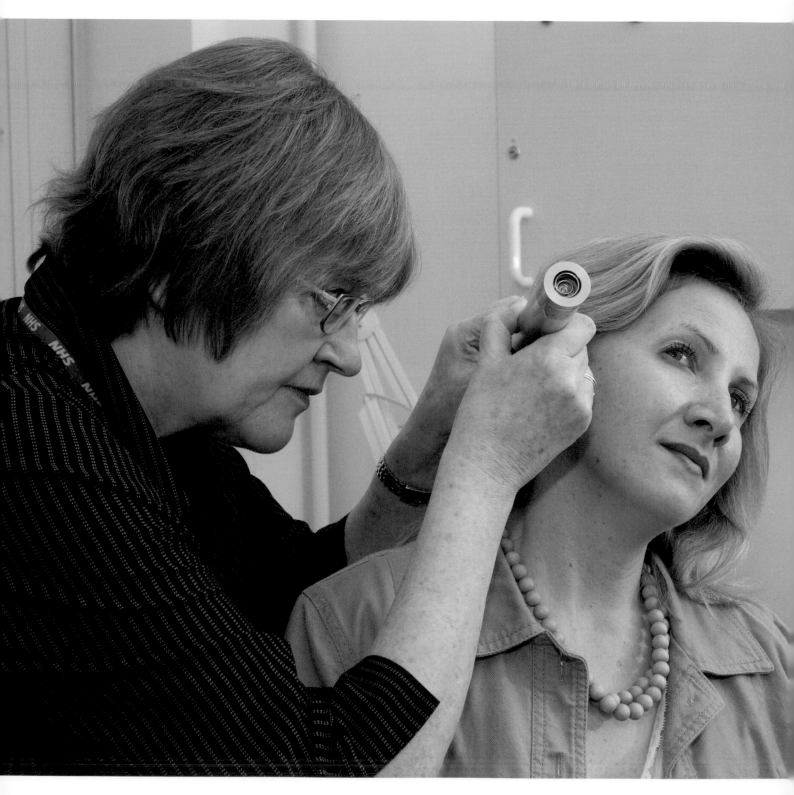

The nurse-practitioner movement challenged existing traditions of health care. Doctors had always "owned" the diagnosis and treatment of patients, with nurses appearing to act as their assistants. Nurse-practitioners, and the doctors they worked with, began to see things differently. For them, the nurse and doctor were equal partners in a patient's care and treatment: their work was a genuine collaboration. The development of the nurse-practitioner movement was rapid and smooth in some regions. This was because, in these areas, physicians were happy to support their nurse-colleagues. In other parts of the country, however, doctors opposed the nurse-practitioner movement and tried to block its development.

The nurse-practitioner movement advanced rapidly in the 1970s, with the help of the federal government and private foundations, which sponsored programs throughout the country. And yet it had had fragile beginnings. The development of new ways of practicing began among a few clinicians in isolated areas, and only really gained ground in the 1980s, when the need for health care cost-savings became more acute. One of the earliest pioneers was Loretta Ford, who with her physician-colleague Henry Silver developed the nurse-practitioner role at the University of Colorado in 1965. Loretta felt that, by developing a nurse-practitioner certificate at the university, she was giving recognition to nurses for work they were already doing. They had, for some time, been working beyond the boundaries of their official role. The nurse-practitioner certificate just confirmed this.

Like so many other reforms that have made a real difference to nursing practice, the nurse-practitioner movement was not imposed on the nursing profession from above (by government or by formal organizations such as the American Nurses' Association), but developed as a fragmented "grassroots" movement. An example of this was the work of Joan Lynaugh and colleagues at the University of Rochester in the late 1960s and early 1970s. Over time, trust developed, doctors and nurses came to work much more closely together, and patients received more thoughtful and knowledgeable care. The nurse's use of clinical judgment was no longer something that happened in secret. It was now a recognized part of her work.

Effects on Nursing Education

The nurse-practitioner movement had a profound effect on nursing education. Up until then, postgraduate level education (master's level) had prepared nurses to be administrators or educators. Nurses could now undertake a higher degree that would prepare them for a particular form of "advanced practice," and would keep them at the bedside. Some believed that the extended knowledge of nurse-practitioners made them something different from other nurses—a hybrid between the doctor and nurse. But nurse-practitioners themselves knew that they were simply being recognized for the knowledge and skills that they already had as nurses. Their knowledge had always overlapped with that of others, such as dieticians, physiotherapists, and counsellors. It was only when their work overlapped with that of the physician that some argued that they were no longer nurses. Yet their expanded scope of practice did not remove the essential nursing skills that were part of their core identity.

Opposite:

Nurse-practitioners have a large repertoire of examination and assessment skills. Here, a nurse-practitioner examines a patient's ear with an otoscope.

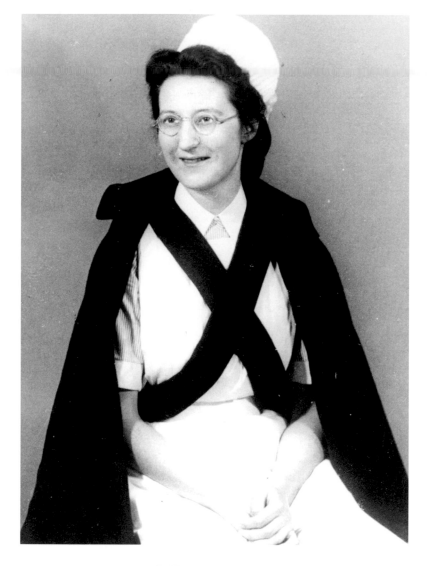

Above:

A portrait of Cicely Saunders. The photograph was taken soon after she qualified as a nurse.

early age. Persuaded by her parents to enter St Anne's College, Oxford, to study philosophy, politics, and economics, she left after a year, interrupting her studies to train as a nurse at St Thomas's Hospital. It was 1940, and Cicely felt she must assist the war effort in some way. Four years later, due to a spinal problem, she was forced to leave nursing, and return to Oxford, where she completed her degree. In 1945, she obtained a diploma in public and social administration and then took a job as an almoner (social worker) at St Thomas's Hospital.

Cicely was inspired to work with the dying by a Jewish-refugee patient named David Tasma. She began to work as a volunteer in various private, charitable homes for the dying, including St Joseph's, a Catholic hospice. She considered establishing an Anglican hospice—a fascinating idea that mirrors the work done by some of the earliest nineteenth-century nurse-reformers. Instead, however, she decided to set up a hospice where individuals of any religion or denomination could feel welcome. She began writing for the medical and nursing press, and drew up a proposal for a hospice in 1959. By this time, Cicely had graduated as a doctor, realizing that a medical qualification would enable her to meet her goals. In 1967, St Christopher's Hospice was opened in London.

Cicely undertook lecture tours—particularly in the USA—and her ideas spread. By the time of her death, 50,000 professionals had trained at the St Christopher's study center, there were about 200 hospices in the UK, and programs had been established in 115 countries of the world. Many thousands of people had read her influential books. She published 85 works in all, including *Living With Dying* (1983). Cicely died in 2005 at St Christopher's Hospice.

THE HOSPICE MOVEMENT

A technological revolution was taking place in health care in the mid-twentieth century. In the middle of this revolution, it was nurses who realized that some patients were being failed. The more money and effort that was expended to keep people alive, the more neglected and isolated were those who could not be saved. Care of the dying became a moral imperative.

Cicely Saunders (1918–2005)

Born on June 22, 1918, in Hertfordshire, England, Cicely Saunders wanted to be a nurse from an

Florence Wald (1917–2008)

The first hospice care program in the USA was founded by Florence Wald in Connecticut, in 1974. Born Florence Sophie Schorske in the Bronx, New York City, on April 19, 1917, Florence was educated at Mount Holyoke College and Yale University. She had been Dean of the School of Nursing at Yale for ten years when, in 1963, she heard an inspirational talk by Cicely Saunders. She decided to devote her life to establishing hospice care in the USA, and resigned from her position at Yale to give herself time to develop her plans. She visited Britain in 1969 to work in St Christopher's Hospice.

After years spent carefully researching the effects of hospice care on patients and their families, Florence Wald developed a home-care program for care of the dying, and then oversaw the development of the first American hospice in Branford, Connecticut. She went on to develop hospice care within the prison services. In the 1980s, the American Medicare system began to pay for hospice care, and the hospice movement became much more widespread, but also more bureaucratic. By the time Florence died, at the age of ninety-one in November 2008, there were more than 3,000 hospice programs in the USA.

Below:
Peg Nelson, a nurse-practitioner at St Joseph Mercy Oakland Hospital, Pontiac, Michigan, talks with patient, Miyoshi Scott.

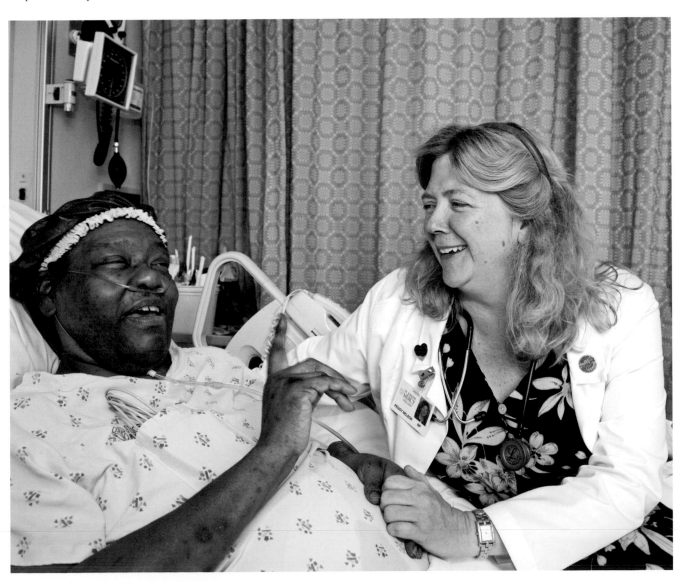

CURE AND CARE

As medicine and surgery became more and more intricate and techniques for keeping people alive advanced, nurses had to become expert technicians. It did not make sense for them to operate complex life-saving machinery "blind," so they became very knowledgeable about what was happening to their patients, before, during, and after treatment. They recognized that their doctor-colleagues were the experts in diagnosis and treatment of disease, but they shared much of that knowledge. They also specialized in understanding how patients responded to illness and treatment, bringing a personal and individual element to the health care of each patient.

As the century progressed, nurses dispelled the myth that they were the doctors' assistants. Instead, it became increasingly clear that the doctor-nurse partnership was a complex one permitting the best possible care to be offered to patients. At the end of the century, patients too became more knowledgeable about their own health, due to advances in education and more readily available knowledge via the World Wide Web. This meant that the educational and supportive roles of the nurse expanded as patients wanted to be aided in being much more directly involved in decisions about their own treatment and care.

Complex treatments such as detailed diagnostic tests, open heart surgery, keyhole surgery, and toxic chemotherapies challenged both doctors and nurses. The more complex a treatment, the greater its potential dangers could be. Some treatments seemed to cause almost as much damage as they repaired, and the extent to which their benefits outweighed their side-effects had to be monitored. This placed nurses at the center of complex ethical decisions about when to begin, continue, or end particular treatments.

One might think that this detailed attention to pathology and physiology would take all the attention of the nurse. But nurses were determined that the more personal and caring elements of their work would not be driven out by their need to attend to more "scientific" principles. Their role continued to be one of carer and comforter, even as the technological elements of their work advanced.

Right:

A nurse examines a baby in a hospital incubator. Neonatal intensive care has become an important area of specialist practice.

Opposite:

The caring elements of nursing remain the bedrock of practice. They depend upon high-level and complex interpersonal skills, which often go unrecognized. As with all artistic work, nursing care is at its best when it is made to look easy.

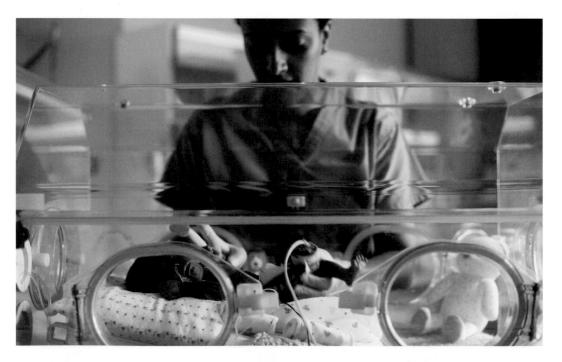

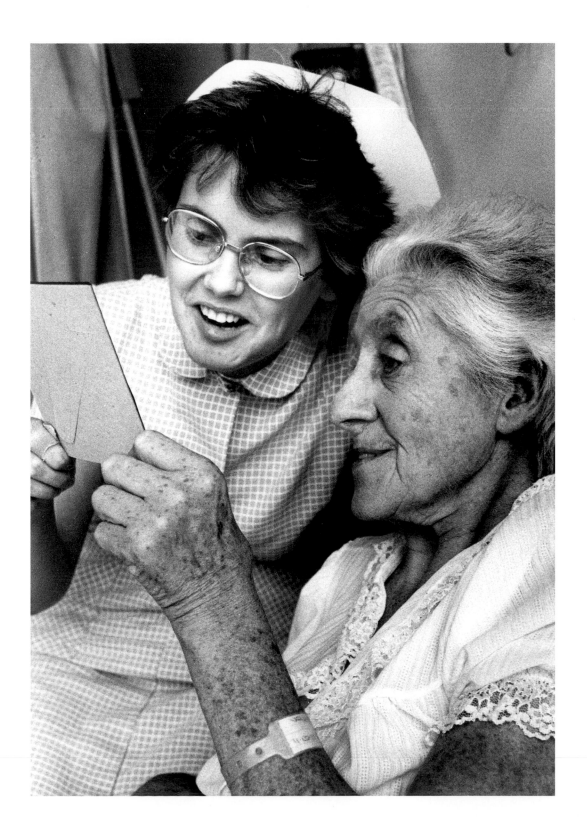

Leaders

There have always been nurses. Yet nursing as a profession and as a discipline has developed only relatively recently. Its emergence was largely due to the energies and abilities of thousands of individual practitioners, but it could not have happened without the drive, inspirational qualities, and assertiveness of important and influential leaders.

Some individuals led by example, and gained public acclaim. Florence Nightingale's important work in the Crimean War could easily have gone unnoticed had it not happened under the intense spotlight of media attention. Nightingale's example, along with her fluent and cogent writings on many subjects, inspired others to join what quickly became an emerging profession. Her messages about the importance of nursing were then carried through the world by individuals such as Lucy Osburn and Alice Fisher. Yet Nightingale herself was inspired by those who had come before her. Important leaders such as Mary Jones and Mary Clare Moore had already kept alive and handed down a legacy which had been developing since earliest times.

Other leaders performed their work through education and research. Adelaide Nutting was the world's first Professor of Nursing and her work created a template for other influential educationalists. In the twentieth century, nursing gained ground rapidly as a discipline, and influential leaders such as Jean McFarlane, Margaret Scott-Wright, and Patricia Benner began to develop theories and educational approaches that would enable the discipline to thrive. One of the most important American educationalists, Virginia Henderson, inspired many nurses by articulating clearly the nature of the work they were doing and by emphasizing its purpose and significance.

Nurses have always found it difficult to influence policy at national and international levels; their status as a predominantly female profession and the apparently menial nature of some of their work has meant that it has been hard for them to find ways into the corridors of power. These societal disadvantages have made all the more extraordinary the efforts of those individuals who have wielded political power. Mrs Bedford Fenwick's agitation for a professional register, and the remarkable efforts of Matrons-in-Chief, such as Maud McCarthy and Hester Maclean, stand as exemplars of nurses' ability to exert influence at the highest levels.

From left to right:
Adelaide Nutting (the world's first Professor of Nursing), Lilian Ward (the founder of public health nursing in the USA), Lucy Osburn (instigator of the Nightingale System in Australia), and Margaret Scott-Wright (the first Professor of Nursing Studies in the UK).

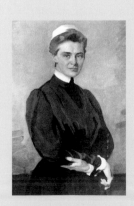 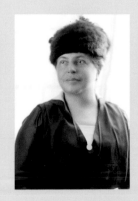 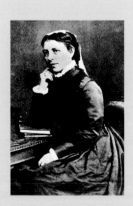 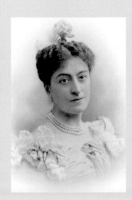

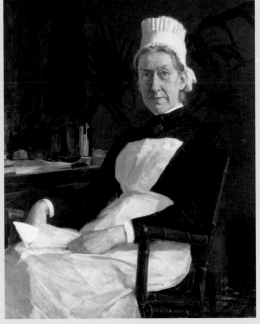

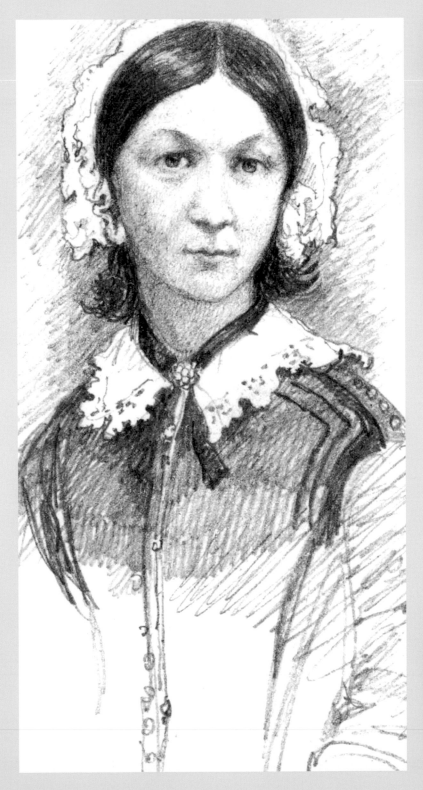

Left:
Florence Nightingale, arguably the world's most famous nurse.

Above:
Alice Fisher, who brought the Nightingale System of Nursing to the USA.

Below:
Virginia Henderson, influential nursing theorist.

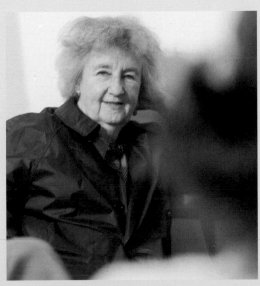

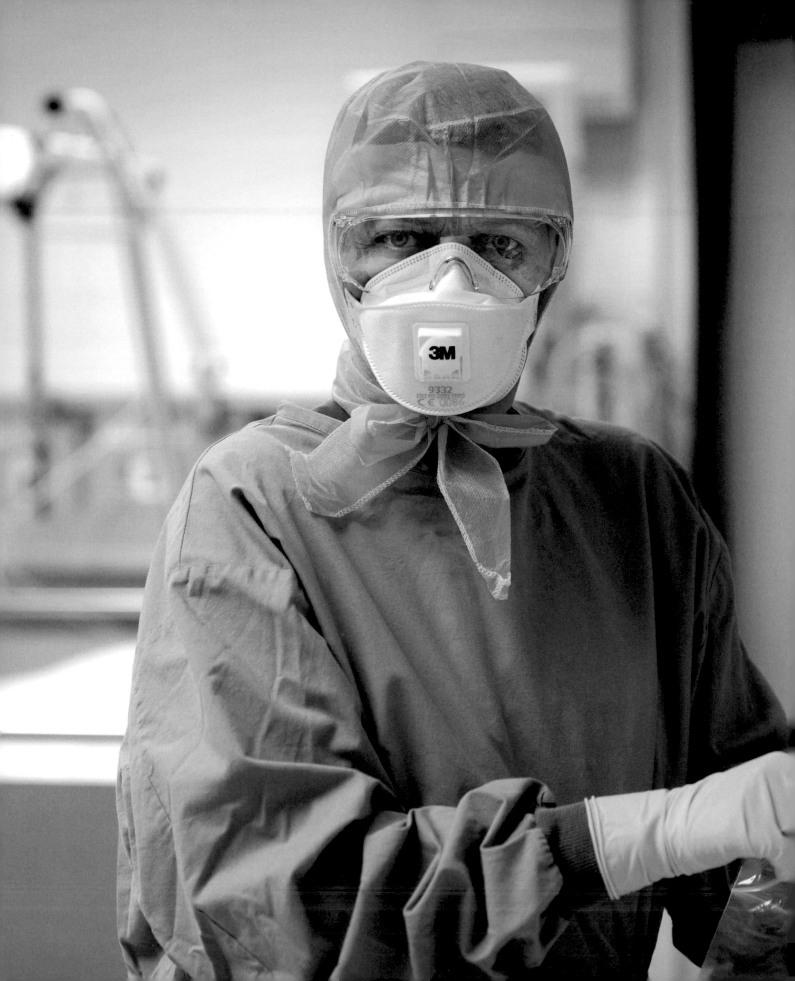

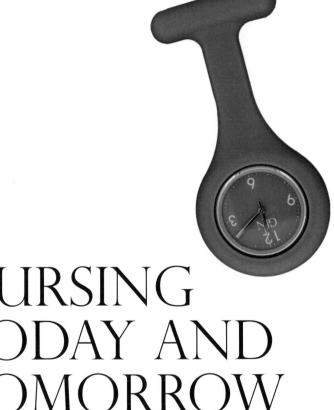

NURSING TODAY AND TOMORROW

4

The new roles for nurses that were established in the late twentieth century are continuing to expand. Four nurses talk about these roles in more detail, offering firsthand insights into their significance.

Nursing in the Twenty-First Century

Previous pages:
Left *A nurse in Frankfurt, Germany, working on the 2009 swine flu outbreak.*

Right *A nurse's fob watch. The silicon cover makes it easy to disassemble and sterilize.*

Nursing practice is advancing rapidly, with the new roles of the late twentieth century continuing to gain strength in spite of economic constraints. Today, nurse specialists in many fields are developing and expanding their practice all over the world, and many advanced practice nurses prescribe a range of medications, run clinics, and perform minor surgery. The increasingly global nature of these roles illustrates how nurses are beginning to recognize their skills and expertise and to find ways of demonstrating their importance to the rest of the world. These nurses owe much to the nurse specialists and nurse-practitioners of the USA, who paved the way for the expansion of nursing practice.

NURSE-PRACTITIONERS IN THE USA

Primarily community-based, nurse-practitioners work with patients who have complex chronic health problems. Working mainly from clinics, they enable patients to manage their problems. They also provide continuity of care when their patients go into and come out of hospital. They need a wide range of expert knowledge, since their duties may include diagnosing complications that arise from illness.

Suzanne Wingate, Adult Nurse-Practitioner in Cardiology

Following a childhood ambition to become a nurse, Suzanne Wingate began her training at the age of eighteen, then worked in the US Navy Nursing Service for twenty-five years, rising from Ensign to Captain. After retiring from the military due to family commitments, she furthered her nursing education, gaining a Masters degree. She then became a clinical specialist, building on work she had done in the Navy with cardiac patients. She gained a doctorate and began to work as a lecturer and researcher, then, realizing that academic work was taking her "further from the patient," she decided to become a nurse-practitioner. She now works as an adult nurse-practitioner (cardiology) for the health agency Kaiser Permanente in Silver Spring, Maryland. Her experience of research has

helped her to develop evidence-based practice in her workplace. She sees herself as "a clinician with an extensive educational background." Suzanne Wingate is now highly influential in the field of Cardiology. She has many publications in academic journals, and is President of the American Association of Heart Failure Nurses, an organization that evolved to work closely with the Heart Failure Society of America. She is a Fellow of the American Heart Association and has been given an award for Clinical Excellence in Nursing by the Heart Failure Society.

"I think that the nurse-practitioner role is becoming more and more powerful, because the current epidemic of chronic illness is just overwhelming, in terms of people living with diabetes, hypertension, heart failure, heart disease, COPD [chronic obstructive pulmonary disease], emphysema—all these chronic illnesses that, for the most part, won't be cured. They're just controlled and managed and a huge amount of lifestyle change, prevention, and management is important to that. These people need regular follow-up and sometimes constant attention and tweaking and adjustments made to their pretty complicated regimens. And I think a nurse-practitioner role is just tailor-made for that, because you have the medical knowledge and the ability legally to prescribe tests, treatments, and medications, and to diagnose, along with the skill of building relationships with patients: being able to

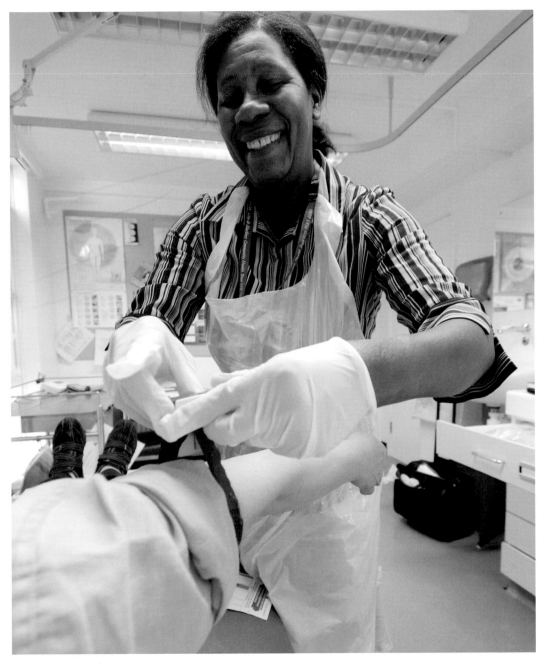

Left:
*A British community
nurse working as part
of the National Health
Service in the borough of
Hackney, in London.*

teach them; being able to follow up; being able to include their family; being able to recognize the psychological factors that are very important in their lives.

"You do sometimes get frustrated when you are not given credit for what you know, or what you've done with the patient, or the abilities you have, just because you're a nurse-practitioner. But when that happens you have to just put your head down and move forward and show by example what you can do… If you know what you're doing you will shine in whatever you do, and the patient will get better.

"I talk to my patients about heart failure being a lot like diabetes. I say: 'We can't cure it, but we're going to control it.' It's a partnership of lifestyle management and medical diagnostic management. It's an illness the patient is going to have for the rest of his or her life, however long that life may be. These patients clearly need the evidence-based medical treatments that are out there, to survive. These treatments have been proven to prolong life and improve quality, so they clearly need that, and as a nurse-practitioner you can prescribe that. But (equally as important) they need to be taught how to manage themselves—how to recognize symptoms; the lifestyle change that's involved, in terms of diet and activity and stress—whatever their particular issues might be. Certainly they need a team, but on that team they need someone who can tune in to the psychosocial issues, the education issues, as well as the medical issues. A nurse-practitioner, by virtue of medical and nursing education, is able to provide all that.

"Also, the role of the nurse-practitioner is a lot more accessible to a patient. Physician schedules or practice-patterns may be such that they don't have the time (or, quite frankly, the knowledge base) to spend talking with the patient about what they need to do in their life. For example, they don't have the time or training to be able to spend twenty minutes of the visit asking questions like "How are you going to go shopping now? I think we are more accessible. We have the meld of medical and nursing knowledge to give patients what they need... For day-to-day long-term management, a nurse-practitioner is the key.

"The power of a nurse should not be underestimated in terms of what we can do for patients when they are so vulnerable. The power we have to help them change their lives—to live longer and feel better—is just immense, and I am not sure all nurses realize that. The father of a friend of mine had some surgery on a heart valve, and she emailed me and two other nurses to say that she had been visiting the hospital for the past week. She said: 'I can't tell you how lucky you are to do what you do. Nurses are the most powerful people in the hospital. I don't think my dad would have done as well as he did without nurses.' That's very rewarding... Nursing is so important. People don't notice us because things tend to run smoothly—and that's because we've made them run smoothly. But people don't always recognize the power of that."

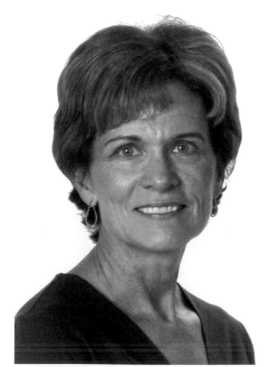

Right:
*A portrait of
Suzanne Wingate.*

Opposite:
*A nurse-practitioner
monitoring a patient's
cardiac test.*

"*The power of a nurse
should not be under-
estimated in terms of what
we can do for patients
when they are so
vulnerable. The power we
have to help them change
their lives ...is just
immense, and I'm not sure
all nurses realize that.*"

Suzanne Wingate

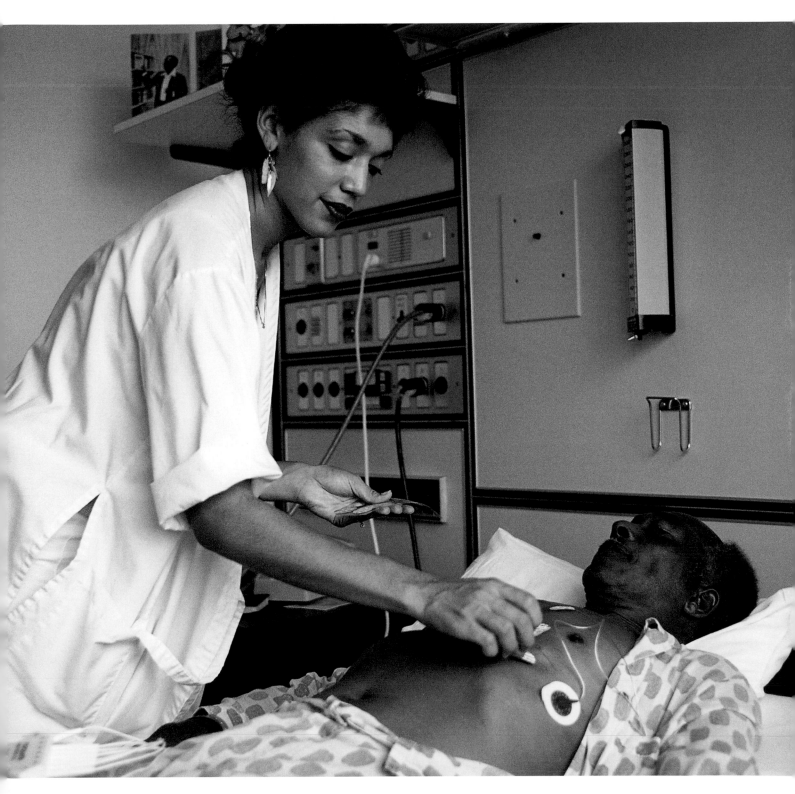

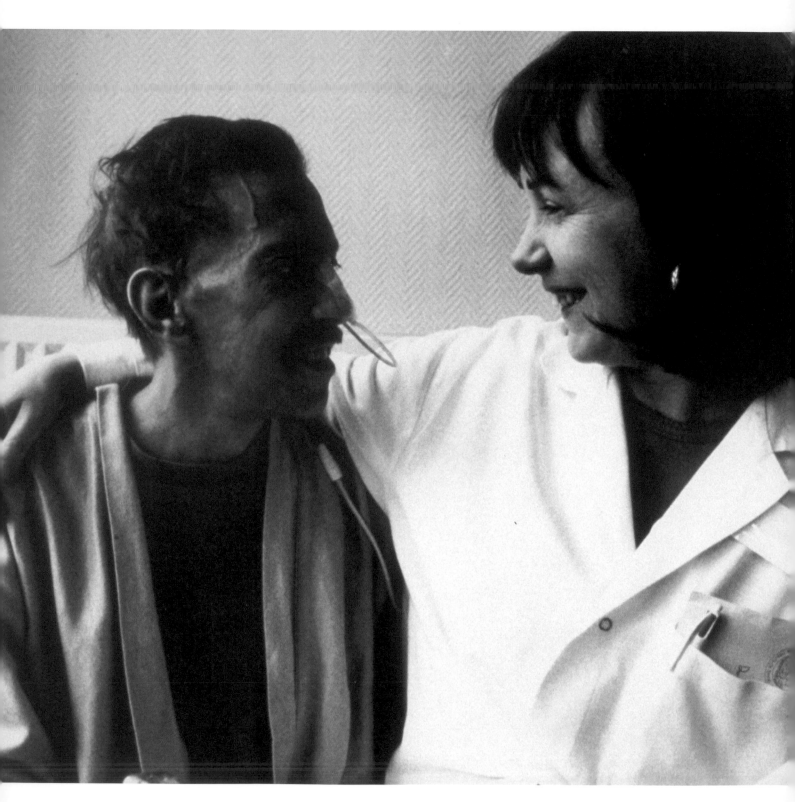

SPECIALIST NURSES

Despite economic restraints and occasional public indifference, the role of the nurse has expanded rapidly over the last two decades throughout the world. In the UK nurses began to develop new, advanced roles in the 1990s, and there is now a range of career options for nurses wishing to develop their practice skills and knowledge.

The role of the "clinical nurse specialist" is becoming increasingly important. It involves working directly with caseloads of patients, offering leadership, support, education, and training to nurse-colleagues and taking a strategic role in the development of services. These high-level nurses have a deep understanding of research in their own fields of practice. They are also able to evaluate the latest technologies. It is these nurses who, in collaboration with doctors, adapt rapidly expanding knowledge and technical advance to make it relevant and useful for patients.

Felicia Cox, Pain Specialist Nurse (UK)

No stranger to the concept of care, as a child Felicia Cox already had experience of caring for a sister with Down Syndrome, and, as the eldest in her family, looked after her siblings. After qualifying as a State Registered Nurse in Tasmania in 1986, she worked in operating-theater nursing for three years in Australia before answering an advertisement in the national press for nurses in Great Britain. In April 1990 she went to work as a theater sister at Harefield Hospital in Buckinghamshire, England, entering the hospital, which, by coincidence, had been run by Australian nurses during the First World War.

Felicia's Australian training meant that she was multiskilled in the operating-theater environment, having experience as a scrub, circulating, recovery, and anesthetic nurse. After working in theaters for seven years, Felicia introduced a new Nurse-Led Pain Service into The Royal Brompton and Harefield Hospitals Trust. In addition to her Australian qualifications, Felicia holds a Masters degree from the University of Westminster.

In April 2005 Felicia discovered she had leukemia and underwent a period of intense illness and hospitalization. She spent six months in one room at St Mary's Hospital, London, receiving chemotherapy and enduring severe side-effects, including a life-threatening fungal lung infection that caused uncontrollable shaking. It was during her time as a patient that she learned firsthand the value of a calm, competent, and caring nurse at her bedside—a nurse who seemed "like a friend." Some of the less experienced nurses seemed "terrified" when she was acutely ill, and she realized that it is only with training and experience that nurses are able to offer the containment and support that patients really need. Although she was already a highly trained and qualified nurse, this experience had a profound influence on Felicia's work, infusing her with a determination to meet her goals—to edit a journal, to write a book, and to complete a PhD.

Opposite:
*A cancer patient
and nurse in Puteaux,
Ile de France.*

Below:
A portrait of Felicia Cox.

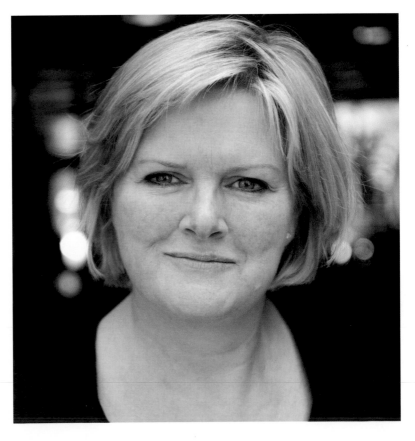

Felicia Cox is now the Clinical Lead for the Cardio-Thoracic Pain Management Service at the Royal Brompton and Harefield Hospitals Trust, UK. She leads a team of four consultant anesthetists, five nurses, and a dedicated pharmacist, with support from physiotherapists and psychologists. She has developed assessment schedules that permit members of her team to accurately assess patients' pain, to document the medications they receive and to monitor their responses to these.

"My move into perioperative care stimulated my desire to understand more about the theory of pain-relief and relate that to practice, so I've evolved the pain management service at Royal Brompton and Harefield into a cutting-edge service. It is very much nurse-led. We are probably unique in the UK, in that a senior nurse is the lead clinician. This role is mostly taken by consultant anesthetists. We offer a limited chronic pain service at Harefield. It's not just perioperative analgesia that we're providing. It's a continuous service throughout the Trust.

"It's well-known that patients can experience persistent pain after surgery. There's lots of evidence to show that if you have poorly managed pain around the time of surgery, then you're much more likely to develop chronic pain. So we take our perioperative analgesia provision very seriously. We tend to use a lot of thoracic epidural analgesia, which is very much a nurse-led service, because my clinical nurses are out there on the wards every day. So because there is a relationship between poorly managed acute pain and chronic pain we do everything we possibly can to reduce the amount of pain that a patient experiences around the time of surgery. Pain isn't just a physical process, it is an emotional process as well, so we spend a lot of time actually providing education to both nurses and patients, be it formal classroom education, lunchtime meetings on specialist topics, or bedside teaching—which I think is where most of our best work is done.

"Having been a patient myself, I used to read and then re-read all of the literature that was given to me, and I thought that a lot of it was in insufficient detail, so I have spent a lot of time in the last two years enhancing the literature that we give patients, explaining to them why it is so important to voice unmanaged pain and any concerns that they have, and the importance of taking regular pain-killers, but also looking out for side-effects that really do affect quality of life such as constipation, which is probably the major reason why people don't take stronger pain-killers. When we think about pain relief and analgesia provision, most people think immediately about reaching for the medicine cabinet. They don't think about listening to what the patient has to say about their pain, and often the patient may be voicing unrelieved pain, but in fact their concerns are anxiety related to disease-progression, or outcome of their surgery, or other sorts of interventions. I would hope that I encourage my nurses to actually sit down and listen and talk to their patients—listen to the patient primarily, and then talk to the patient and identify whether it is in fact unrelieved pain they are experiencing or something else. My nurses are able to understand the emotional, sensory, and physical processes their patients are experiencing, and I think that ability to see the whole picture is unique to nurses.

"Pharmacists are very much geared toward medicines, interventions, interactions; and doctors are very much interested in the state of the patient seen while standing at the end of the bed. But pain is a subjective experience. You can stand by a patient's bedside and ask them to take a deep breath in and have a cough, and watch out for grimacing or look for physiological signs that they may be experiencing pain, such as high blood pressure or increased pulse rate, but it's the patient's experience that's important. There is no objective measure of how much pain they are experiencing, so I think nursing is very important. And I also think that, being a nurse, we have, probably, enhanced communication skills compared to other disciplines.

"I consider myself to be the champion—I am always trying to drive things forward—to develop the services. I also develop my team and I actively encourage interdisciplinary learning and mutual support."

Patricia Davidson: Professor of Cardiovascular and Chronic Care (Australia)

One of an increasing number of nurses who have combined specialist nursing with academic work, Patricia Davidson had been studying Arts and Political Sciences in the mid-1970s at university, when she decided to discontinue her course and go into nursing. After training from 1977 to 1980 in

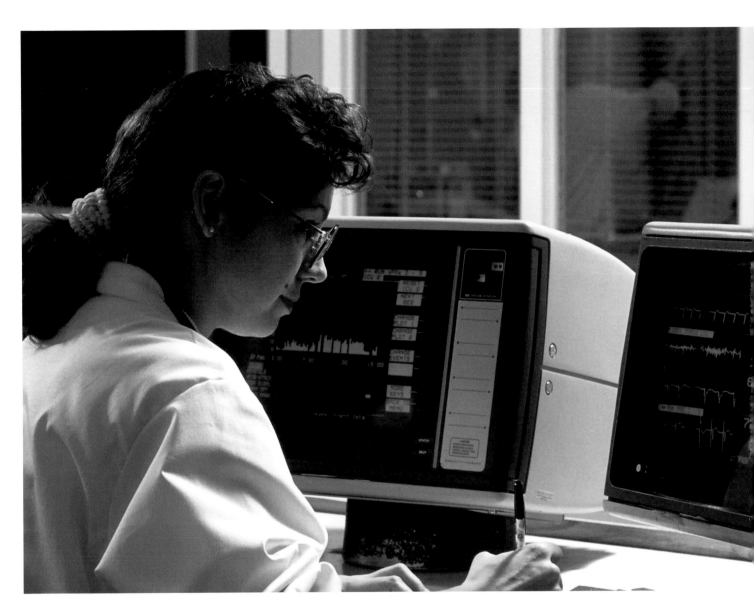

Wollongong, south of Sydney, she moved to Sydney itself, where she underwent further training in intensive care nursing and remained in that field.

In the mid-1980s, Patricia decided she would like to move into nursing education, and worked for a time as a clinical educator in a demonstration program. Her grueling schedule involved spending half of her time in the hospital and half in the university. After moving back into practice for about seven years, she became a Research Nurse in Heart Failure Care in Sydney. Here, she worked with an inspiring physician-mentor, who recognized her talent and encouraged her to embark on PhD-level studies.

Patricia completed her PhD in 2002 and developed a clinical and academic career. She is now Professor of Cardiovascular and Chronic Care at Curtin University of Technology and the Professorial Chair in Cardiovascular Nursing Research at St Vincent's and Mater Health in Sydney.

Above:

A nurse at a cardiac monitoring station.

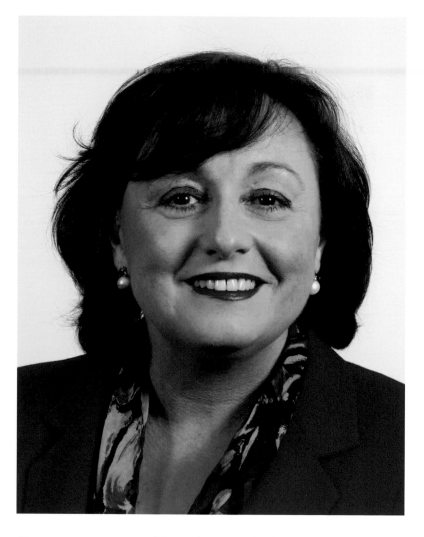

Above:

A portrait of Patricia Davidson.

facilitate a good death is a very rewarding experience, but it only comes with training, experience, and exploration of your own feelings about death and dying.

"In the course of their work, nurses have huge exposure to death and dying. Palliative care is an enormously important area of practice and one that has been recognized for some time in cancer care. In areas such as heart-failure, respiratory disease, diabetes, dementia, and a whole range of other illnesses it is only now beginning to be recognized, and nurses are at the forefront of the development of what is an exciting and crucial area of care—particularly in the context of a global epidemic of chronic diseases and an aging population.

"A dignified death should be a basic human right. Yet, in the midst of technological innovation, where we live in a death-defying society and prize longevity at all costs, this is not always the case. Nurses are in the best position to ensure that this right is maintained and can minimize suffering for both patients and their families, by promoting adequate symptom management, providing support, and facilitating effective communication."

CASE MANAGERS IN THE UK

One of the newest innovations in the UK is the case manager. Along with the community matron, the case manager has a wide remit within community-settings to care for individuals with complex long-term illnesses. Some patients will have many diseases occurring simultaneously, and will be taking a complex "cocktail" of drugs that has to be carefully monitored. British case managers are very similar to the nurse-practitioners of the USA. They coordinate proactive health and social care for individuals with severe chronic illnesses who are "high-intensity users" of the health services. They attend Masters-level courses, which include training in high-level clinical skills such as full physical assessments. They do much of the work that would previously have been done only by general medical practitioners; but this does not make them doctors. Their broad-ranging nurse-training, which gave them skills and knowledge in the physical, emotional, and social care of their patients, is brought into play in helping them to support and empower society's most vulnerable members.

"Nurses play a critical role in supporting patients and their families in periods of transition. One of the most vulnerable periods for patients and their families is when they have to face death—particularly in an illness where they have reached the brink of death several times and survived. What people fear most is not death itself but the process of dying. Nurses can play a crucial part in alleviating suffering and offering support to patients and their families at this time.

"Suffering is not only physical. Nurses can relieve pain and other distressing symptoms. But their work goes much further than this. They also help patients address their existential and spiritual suffering. They can do this independently or collaboratively as part of a team. To

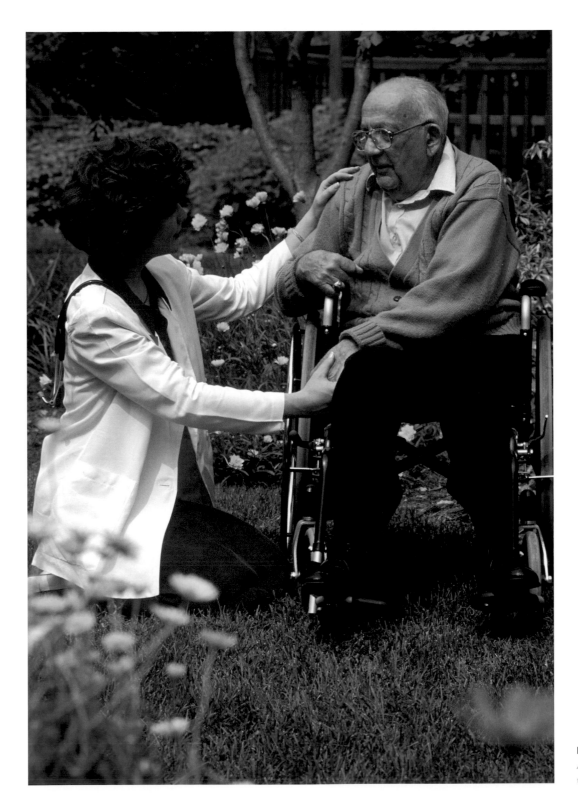

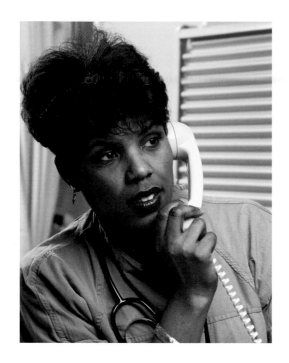

Right:
An American nurse-practitioner.

NURSE CONSULTANTS

One of the most important nursing roles to develop in the UK is that of the nurse consultant, a role that epitomizes the ways in which nurses are taking control of their own areas of expertise.

Usually, though not exclusively, hospital-based nurse consultants use their specialist knowledge to treat patients with specific health conditions. They also teach and advise their nursing colleagues. Like nurse-practitioners, they offer continuity of care, remaining with the same patients for long periods of time.

Karen Clancy: Nurse Consultant (UK)

British nurse Karen Clancy qualified as a State Enrolled Nurse (SEN, the lower of two tiers of qualification in the UK at that time) in 1984, after having taken a break in the middle of her training to have her first child. The mid-1980s was a time of economic crisis in the UK, and jobs for nurses were scarce. It was to be some time before she found a job—in the Royal Oldham, the hospital where she had trained. She worked for some years on the night shift, caring for patients on a number of different general medical and surgical wards.

At this point, Karen realized that, if she wanted to advance her career, she must become a Registered General Nurse (RGN, the highest basic qualification offered in the UK at that time). She therefore embarked on the tough and demanding "conversion course," juggling family commitments (she now had two young children) with work and study. During her course she witnessed a tragic death that changed her thinking and transformed her life. A very young woman whose breast cancer had not been diagnosed early enough was dying in a hospital side-ward. The woman was distraught because she was not able to see her children once more before she died. There was a photograph of the children on the bedside locker, and Karen placed it on the woman's chest and closed her hands around it, saying, "Your children are with you now." In that moment, Karen realized the importance of health education. She went on to spend time working in the community and in preventive care, doing whatever she could to enable and empower people to live the best and most healthy lives possible. In the impoverished, deprived populations of the Lancashire mill towns, people were living "against the odds," and needed nurses who would act as their advocates and supporters.

Some months after qualifying, Karen took a job in general practice, working as a "practice nurse" and developing services in the community. The role was at that time a new one, which gave Karen the autonomy she needed. She was offered a full-time post running clinics for patients with long-term chronic conditions such as heart disease, diabetes, and asthma. She began to develop a special interest in patients with respiratory diseases.

Karen began to realize that her skills and knowledge were outstripping the obvious boundaries of her role as an asthma nurse, and in 2000, as the role of "nurse consultant" began to emerge in the UK, she took advantage of the offer to apply to become Rochdale's Respiratory Nurse Consultant. During her interview, she gave a presentation, using Patricia Benner's theory of developing from "novice to expert" (see page 121) in explaining how nurses' skills and knowledge could move forward. Some years later, the Chief Executive was to inform her that he often referred to her in after-dinner speeches. For him, she was an inspirational nurse: "You started as an SEN and look where you are now!" he told her.

Karen was the second Respiratory Nurse Consultant to be appointed in England, and soon discovered that other nursing staff—both in hospital and in the community—saw her as a natural leader, and as someone with vast specialist knowledge: someone they could turn to for help and advice. She helped nurses to expand their roles, and to fight the prevailing assumption that they simply followed "medical orders." She encouraged them to have confidence in their own skills of assessment and treatment. At this time, she decided to embark on PhD-level studies, becoming Dr Karen Clancy in 2007. Her PhD, she believed, made her a much better nurse by developing both her listening skills and her analytical abilities.

Soon after taking on the role of nurse consultant, Karen worked with her Primary Care Trust to negotiate the funding for a Respiratory Home Care Service, which enabled patients to be discharged from hospital earlier than might previously have been possible, offering support that would allow them to stay in their own homes.

Since 2007, Karen has been working for Heywood, Middleton and Rochdale Primary Care Trust. She is now Nurse Consultant Long Term Conditions, and manages a team of three community matrons, fifteen case managers, and one pharmacist.

"Being a nurse consultant is about leadership, about being strategic, about auditing activity and about research and development. I have always been strategic in my approach, and I have always had a good relationship with medics. When I was Respiratory Nurse Consultant for Rochdale, I would follow patients from hospital to community and, if necessary, back again. There are many advanced roles for nurses now. The most significant are the 'specialists,' the 'practitioners,' and the 'consultants.' Of these three, the consultant role is

the one that involves the most strategic leadership ...A nurse consultant has a holistic view of the patient. She has specialist knowledge, backed-up by extra training. My training has made me a better nurse, not just by giving me more skills and knowledge, but also by giving me the authority and autonomy to make decisions that I would otherwise have had to ask a medic to make. I don't want—and have never wanted—to be a doctor, but being a nurse consultant means that my nursing knowledge and nursing skills are fully respected for what they are. When I first took on the role, I suddenly realized that I wasn't really doing anything very different from what I had done before. I had been working at that level before I was given the title, but the title gave me the recognition I needed. The PhD was also important. It made me a better nurse—a better listener. The experience of interviewing patients for my study and really listening to what they had to say was very powerful. And now I am managing a number of advanced practitioners.

"People living with long term conditions have still got a life to live. We respect them as the individuals they are and offer them the help they want in their own homes. We also support their carers. Our aim is to help people achieve independence and live as fulfilling lives as possible."

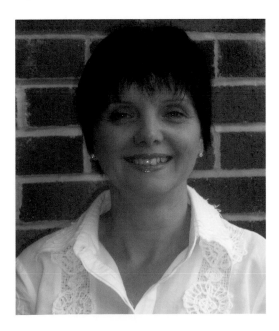

Left:
A portrait of Karen Clancy.

CONCLUSION

As practitioner, specialist, and consultant roles develop throughout the world, individual highly trained nurses at the grassroots level ensure that these roles remain relevant and useful for patients, never losing sight of their inheritance in a nursing profession that has been involved in care, cure, and healing for millennia.

The work of nurses such as Suzanne Wingate, Felicia Cox, Patricia Davidson, and Karen Clancy has evolved out of a long tradition that extends back to ancient times. A nurse practitioner like Suzanne Wingate can trace her inheritance back to the Henry Street Settlement and the ground-breaking work of Lillian Wald (see page 74). The knowledgeable and highly strategic approaches of pain specialists like Felicia Cox have grown out of the detailed work of generations of hospital nurses. Those individuals who developed "surgical nursing" as a specialism in the late nineteenth century were laying the foundations for a world in which nurses such as Felicia could lead teams of clinical specialists. Academic specialists like Patricia Davidson are building on the work of pioneers such as Cicely Saunders and Florence Wald (see page 160). We can trace a direct lineage from the extraordinary work of Karen Clancy with deprived communities in the north of England, to the District Nursing Associations of the nineteenth century (see page 70), and even further to the European tertiary orders of the Medieval and Early Modern worlds (see page 18).

Nurses continue to work on the front lines in the most dangerous scenarios. They accompany troops to war-zones, aid-workers to areas of famine and deprivation, and public health workers to centers of epidemic disease. They are at the forefront of efforts throughout the world to control outbreaks of new killer-microbes, and to contain and heal the devastating trauma inflicted by terrorist attack.

At the same time, nurses are continuing to develop the artistry of their core practice. It is they who are responsible for the most detailed and intricate care of helpless and vulnerable patients. In maintaining and developing their fundamental core skills, nurses are keeping alive a tradition that extends back to the work of healers in the earliest known civilizations.

What is striking about today's nurses is the enormous scope and breadth of their practice. Not only do they pay attention to the most fundamental needs of their patients: the need for cleanliness; for nutritious food and adequate fluids; for a calm, quiet, clean environment; they also prescribe drugs and use sophisticated technologies. They lead teams of clinicians that include nurses, doctors, and other health-care workers. They make strategic decisions about how to adequately meet the health needs of whole populations.

Today's nurses are carers, healers, technicians, decision-makers, and high-level political thinkers. Their story is not a simple one of "progress." It has more to do with endurance and adaptation. In every era, nurses have developed their practice to suit the times. When there have been epidemics and wars, nurses have been there to contain them. When there has been a rapid technological expansion, nurses have adapted new treatments to the needs of patients. Where cure has been possible, nurses have given the necessary treatments, and where death was inevitable, nurses have steered their patients through its trials, giving comfort and care. They have kept alive the knowledge, skills, wisdom, and practices that have made them the world's greatest healers.

Right:
*Nurse Katelyn Carey at her 2009
graduation pinning ceremony at Biola
University, California. The symbolic
welcome of newly graduated nurses
into the nursing profession, pinning
ceremonies (in which nurses are
presented with a pin by their nursing
faculty), are still carried out in many
training schools.*

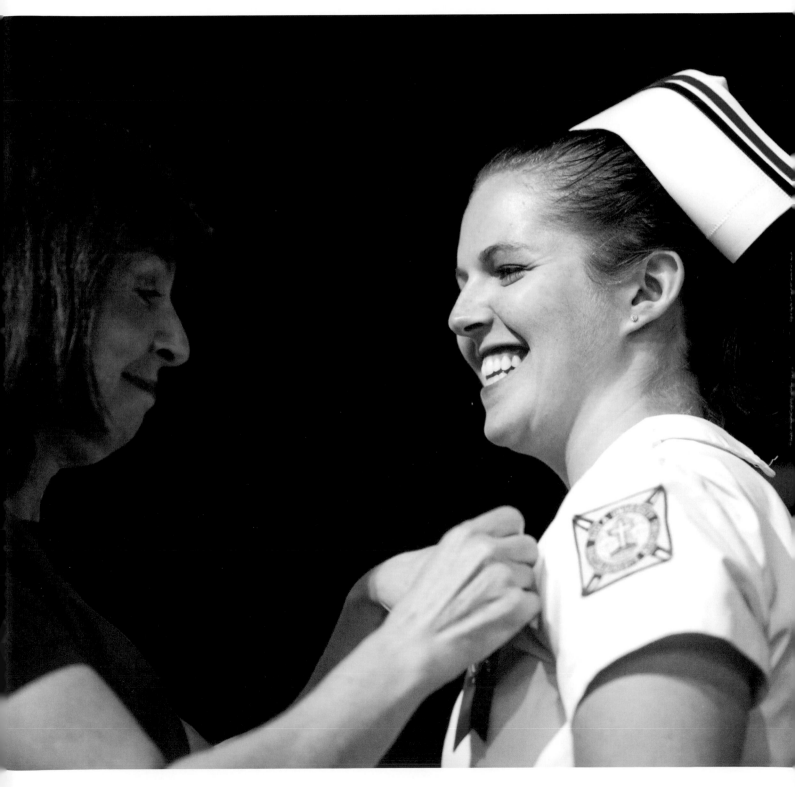

Heroes

Nursing work is, by its very nature, heroic. It is not possible to be an effective nurse without engaging with the physical damage and emotional distress of patients. This ability to engage without being destroyed is the most extraordinary element of nursing expertise; it is also the least visible and the least appreciated. Through millennia of experience, nurses working with suffering and vulnerable people have handed down, from expert to novice, their understanding of how to offer real help to patients without themselves succumbing to despair: that is their art.

Some individual nurses have exhibited an almost superhuman heroism in the course of their work. From the Black Death to modern infectious diseases, and in wars, terrorist attacks, and natural disaster zones, nurses have put themselves at risk to save others. Nurses have taken health care to remote and dangerous territories. Jeanne Mance braved the wild winters and the dangerous conflicts of early-modern Quebec to bring expert nursing care to her fellow-pioneers. Edith Cavell faced death rather than betray those who came to her for help. Mary Breckinridge overcame her own despair at the tragic loss of her children to create an extraordinary organization, the Frontier Nursing Service, which offered health advice and nursing care to the poorest and most deprived American settlers.

Other individuals, while less obviously brave in the physical sense, have exhibited a remarkable courage in the face of adversity. Nurses have been at the forefront of the fight against cultural prejudice, acting as advocates to patients of every race and religion. In the nineteenth and early twentieth centuries, many wore the Red Cross to denote that they would help friend and "enemy" alike. Mary Eliza Mahoney stands as an example of a nurse who represented the fight against racial prejudice. The first African American registered nurse, she was an important participant in the fight to establish career opportunities for minorities. From caring for the dying and traumatized without flinching, to facing death, injury, and disease themselves, nurses all over the world have demonstrated humanity and courage: qualities at the heart of their identity.

From left to right:
British nurse Edith Cavell (who died saving soldiers in the First World War); American nurse Mary Eliza Mahoney (who fought racial prejudice to become the first African American registered nurse); French nurse Jeanne Mance (who braved danger to bring nursing care to European settlements in Canada); and British nurse Jan Pilgrim (who was awarded a nursing Royal Red Cross in 2008 for her work on the front line in Iraq).

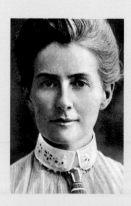 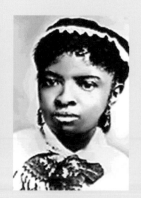 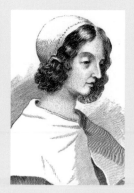 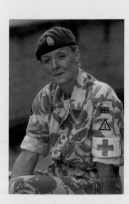

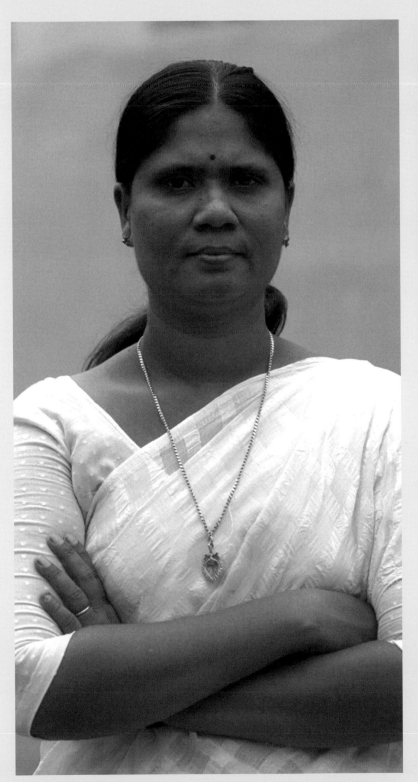

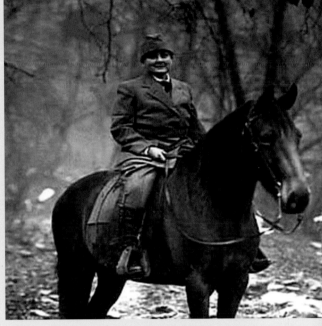

Left:
Nirmala Palsamy, head of the Village Health Nurse Association in Tamil Nadu State, was named by Time Magazine in 2000 as one of the Heroes of the Planet, for her work on family planning in India.

Above:
Mary Breckinridge, founder of the Frontier Nursing Service.

Below:
French Air Force Nurse Genevieve De Galard-Terraube shaking hands with President Eisenhower after being presented with the Medal of Freedom for her service in the Korean War.

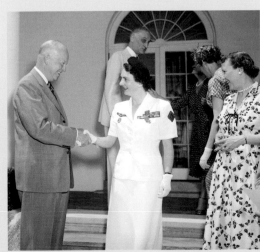

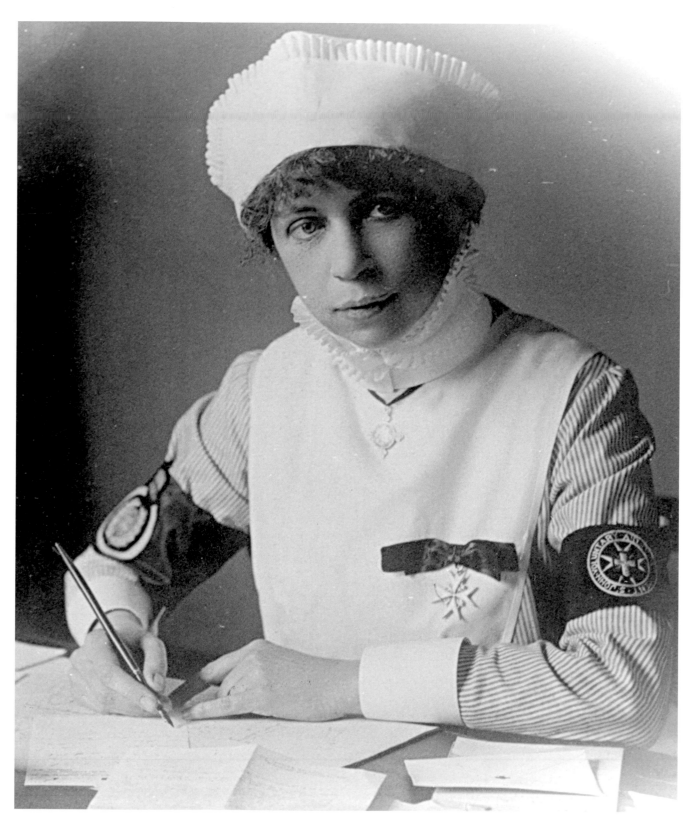

Bibliography

Abel-Smith, Brian, *A History of the Nursing Profession* (Heinemann Educational Books, London 1960)

Baly, Monica, *Florence Nightingale and the Nursing Legacy,* Second Edition (Whurr Publishers Ltd, London 1997)

Bates, Christina; Dodd, Dianne; Rousseau, Nicole (eds), *On All Frontiers: Four Centuries of Canadian Nursing,* (University of Ottawa Press/Canadian Museum of Civilization, Ottawa 2005)

Benner, Patricia, *From Novice to Expert: Excellence and Power in Clinical Nursing Practice* (Addison-Wesley, Menlo Park, CA, 1984)

Bostridge, Mark, *Florence Nightingale. The Woman and Her Legend* (Viking, London 2008)

Buhler-Wilkerson, Karen, *No Place Like Home. A History of Nursing and Home Care in the United States* (The Johns Hopkins University Press, Baltimore 2001)

D'Antonio, Patricia; Baer, Ellen; Rinker, Sylvia; Lynaugh, Joan, *Nurses' Work. Issues Across Time and Place* (Springer Publishing Company, New York 2007)

Diack, Lesley, *Labrador Nurse* (Victor Gollancz Ltd, London 1963)

Dock, Lavinia, L., *A History of Nursing. The Evolution of Nursing Systems from the Earliest Times to the Foundation of the First English and American Training Schools for Nurses,* Volumes III and IV (G. P. Putnam's Sons, New York and London 1912)

Donahue, Patricia, *Nursing, The Finest Art,* Second Edition (Mosby, St Louis 1996)

Elliott, Jayne, "Blurring the Boundaries of Space: Shaping Nursing Lives at the Red Cross Outposts in Ontario, 1922–1945," *Canadian Bulletin of Medical History,* 21, 2, 303–325.

Eva, Sister, *Scenes in the Life of a Nurse* (Bembrose and Sons, London 1890)

Evans, Jonathan, *Edith Cavell* (The Royal London Hospital Museum, London 2008)

Fairman, Julie, and Lynaugh, Joan, *Critical Care Nursing: A History* (University of Pennsylvania Press, Philadelphia 1998)

Fairman, Julie, *Making Room in the Clinic. Nurse Practitioners and the Evolution of Modern Health Care* (Rutgers University Press, New Brunswick 2008)

Gibbon, John Murray, in collaboration with Mathewson, Mary S., *Three Centuries of Canadian Nursing* (The MacMillan Company, Toronto 1947)

Goodnow, Minnie, *Outlines of Nursing History* (W. B Saunders, Philadelphia 1923)

Gordon, Suzanne, *Nursing Against the Odds* (Cornell University Press, Ithaca 2005)

Gordon, Suzanne, *Life Support. Three Nurses on the Front Lines* (Cornell University Press, Ithaca 2007; first published by Little, Brown and Company, 1997)

Hallam, Julia, *Nursing The Image. Media, Culture and Professional Identity* (Routledge, London 2000)

Henderson, Virginia, *The Nature of Nursing: A Definition and its Implications for Practice, Research, and Education* (Macmillan, New York 1966)

Howse, Carrie, *Rural District Nursing in Gloucestershire, 1880–1925* (Reardon Publishing, Cheltenham, Gloucestershire, 2008)

Kalisch, Philip, and Kalisch, Beatrice, *The Changing Image of the Nurse* (Addison Wesley Publishing Company, Menlo Park, CA, 1987)

Kalisch, Philip, and Kalisch, Beatrice, *American Nursing. A History,* Fourth Edition (Lippincott, Williams and Wilkins, Philadelphia 2004)

Keeling, Arlene, *Nursing and the Privilege of Prescription* (Ohio State University Press, Columbus 2007)

Luckes, Eva, *General Nursing,* Second Edition (Kegan Paul, Trench, Trubner and Co., London 1884)

Lynaugh, Joan, and Brush, Barbara, *American Nursing: From Hospital to Health Systems* (Blackwood Press, Cambridge, MA, 1996)

Manton, Jo, *Sister Dora* (Methuen, New York 1971)

McBryde, Brenda, *A Nurse's War* (Chatto and Windus, London 1979)

McBryde, Brenda, *Quiet Heroines. Nurses of the Second World War* (Chatto and Windus, London 1985)

McGann, Susan, *The Battle of the Nurses* (Scutari Press, London 1992)

McPherson, Kathryn, *Bedside Matters. The Transformation of Canadian Nursing, 1900-1990* (University of Toronto Press, Toronto 2003; first published by Oxford University Press Canada, 1996)

Nelson, Sioban, *Say Little, Do Much, Nursing, Nuns and Hospitals in the Nineteenth Century* (University of Pennsylvania Press, Philadelphia 2001)

Nightingale, Florence, *Notes on Nursing. What it is and What it is Not* (Churchill Livingstone, Edinburgh 1980; first published by Harrison and Sons, 1859)

Norris, Rachel, *Norris's Nursing Notes. Being a Manual of Medical and Surgical Information for the use of Hospital Nurses and Others* (Sampson Low, Marston and Co., Ltd, London 1891)

Nutting, M. Adelaide, and Dock, Lavinia L., *A History of Nursing. The Evolution of Nursing Systems from the Earliest Times to the Foundation of the First English and American Training Schools for Nurses,* Volumes I and II (G. P. Putnam's Sons, New York and London 1907)

Piggott, Juliet, *Queen Alexandra's Royal Army Nursing Corps* (Leo Cooper Ltd, London 1975)

Priestley, Susan, *Bush Nursing in Victoria, 1910–1975. The First 75 Years* (Lothian Publishing Company, Melbourne 1986)

Rafferty, Anne Marie, *The Politics of Nursing Knowledge* (Routledge, London 1996)

Richards, Linda, *America's First Trained Nurse* (Diggory Press, Liskeard, UK, 2006)

Schultz, Bartz, *A Tapestry of Service. The Evolution of Nursing in Australia. Volume I: Foundation to Federation, 1788–1900* (Churchill Livingstone, Melbourne 1991)

Seymer, Lucy R., *A General History of Nursing* (Faber and Faber Ltd, London 1949)

Stein, Leonard, "The Doctor–Nurse Game," *Archives of General Psychiatry,* 16, 6, 699–703 (1967)

Stewart, Isla, and Cuff, Herbert E., *Practical Nursing,* Four Volumes (William Blackwood, Edinburgh 1899–1903

Stocks, Mary, *A Hundred Years of District Nursing* (Allen and Unwin, London 1960)

Summers, Anne, *Angels and Citizens. British Women as Military Nurses, 1854–1914,* Revised Edition (Threshold Press, Newbury, Berks., 2000)

Sweet, Helen, with Dougal, Rona, *Community Nursing and Primary Healthcare in Twentieth-Century Britain* (Routledge, London 2007)

Taylor, Eric, *Wartime Nurse. One Hundred Years from the Crimea to Korea 1854–1954* (Robert Hale, London 2001)

Thurstan, Violetta, *Field Hospital and Flying Column: Being the Journal of an English Nursing Sister* (G. P. Putnam's Sons, London 1915)

Tomey, Ann Marriner, and Alligood, Martha Raile, *Nursing Theorists and Their Work,* Fifth Edition (Mosby, St Louis 2002)

Addresses and websites

USA

American Museum of Nursing
300 East Curry Road
Community Services Building
Tempe, AZ 85287
http://asu.edu/museums/oc/nursing.htm

The museum portrays the image of the nurse through the years, from the handmaidens of the early-to-mid 1800s, to the Angels of the 1900s, the "Husband Hunters" of the 1950s, and, finally, today's professional nurses.

Barbara Bates Center for the Study of the History of Nursing
University of Pennsylvania
School of Nursing, Nursing Education Building
Philadelphia, PA 19104-9959
www.nursing.upenn.edu/history

The center was established in 1985 to encourage and facilitate historical scholarship on health-care history and nursing in the United States and across the globe. The center is open to researchers by appointment.

Center for Nursing Historical Inquiry at the University of Virginia
McLeod Hall
202 Jeanette Lancaster Way
Charlottesville, VA 22903
www.nursing.virginia.edu/contact

The Center for Norsing Historical Inquiry is dedicated to the preservation and study of nursing history in the United States. The archive holds extensive collections of manuscripts and photographs.

Clendening History of Medicine Library and Museum
1020–1030 Robinson Building
University of Kansas Medical Center campus
Kansas City, Kansas
http://clendening.kumc.edu

The library collects rare books as well as current works in the history of medicine, nursing, and the allied professions. Under the auspices of its museum, the library also owns hundreds of medical artefacts.

History of Medicine Division, National Library of Medicine
8600 Rockville Pike
Bethesda, MD 20894
http://nlm.nih.gov./hmd

The National Library of Medicine manuscript collection includes the American College of Nurse Midwives, the Henry Street Settlement, the National Organization for Public Health Nursing, the Society of Superintendents of Training Schools, the National League for Nursing Education, and the National League for Nursing.

Maryland School of Nursing Museum
655 W. Lombard Street
Baltimore, MD 21201
www.nursing.umaryland.edu/about/campus-community/museum

Permanent museum exhibition and archives documenting the evolution of Maryland's largest and oldest continuously operated school of nursing from its founding as a hospital training school in 1889 to a leading research institution.

Midwest Nursing History Research Center at the University of Illinois, Chicago
845 S. Damen Ave.
Chicago, IL 60612-7350
www.uic.edu/nursing/ghlo/resourcecenter/index.shtml

The Midwest Nursing History Resource Center maintains a museum with nursing-related artefacts.

The Museum of Nursing History
761 Sproul Road, #299
Springfield, PA 19064
www.nursinghistory.org

The museum is a repository in which individuals can place priceless memorabilia—books, documents, letters, photographs, scrapbooks, yearbooks, caps and uniforms , medals, pins, and military artefacts.

Sea View Hospital Healthcare Museum
460 Brielle Avenue
Staten Island
New York
10314
www.seaviewmuseum.org

The Sea View Hospital Healthcare Museum depicts nine stations full of health-care memorabilia dating as far back as 1881. The museum offers historical classroom presentations on the impact of tuberculosis on the nation from 1910 to 1960. A curriculum on tuberculosis and Sea View's role in its cure is distributed to each class prior to its scheduled tour.

CANADA

Associated Medical Services Nursing History Research Unit at the University of Ottawa
451 Smyth Road
Ottawa, ON K1H 8M5
www.health.uottawa.ca/nursinghistory

The unit is the first formal research unit in Canada dedicated to the history of nursing.

Belleville General Hospital
Online museum
www.bghmuseum.com

History of Belleville General Hospital through a picture library of memoirs, uniforms, medical artefacts, and other documents.

Musée des Hospitalières de l'Hôtel-Dieu de Montreal
201 Avenue des Pins Ouest
Montreal, Quebec H2W 1R5
www.museedeshospitalieres.qc.ca

Located next to the Hôtel-Dieu Hospital, this museum tells the story of the foundation of Montreal and of the exceptional life of Jeanne Mance. Although not a member of the order, she led the work of cloistered nuns who tended the sick in early Montreal beginning in 1644.

Museum of Health Care
Ann Baillie Building
Kingston General Hospital
George St
Kingston, Ontario K7L 2V7
www.museumofhealthcare.ca

More than 27,000 artefacts have been acquired, of which 13,000 are fully accessioned. The museum sponsors displays on site, outreach galleries in the Kingston health care community, and outreach education programs, and is also open for visits.

Nursing History Resource Centre
Nurses Association of New Brunswick
165 Regent Street
Fredericton, N. B. E3B 7B4
www.nanb.nb.ca

The Nursing History Resource Centre was established in July 1992 through the initial support of the Nurses Association of New Brunswick. The Centre, custodian for New Brunswick's past, has an exhibit area and an adjoining archive.

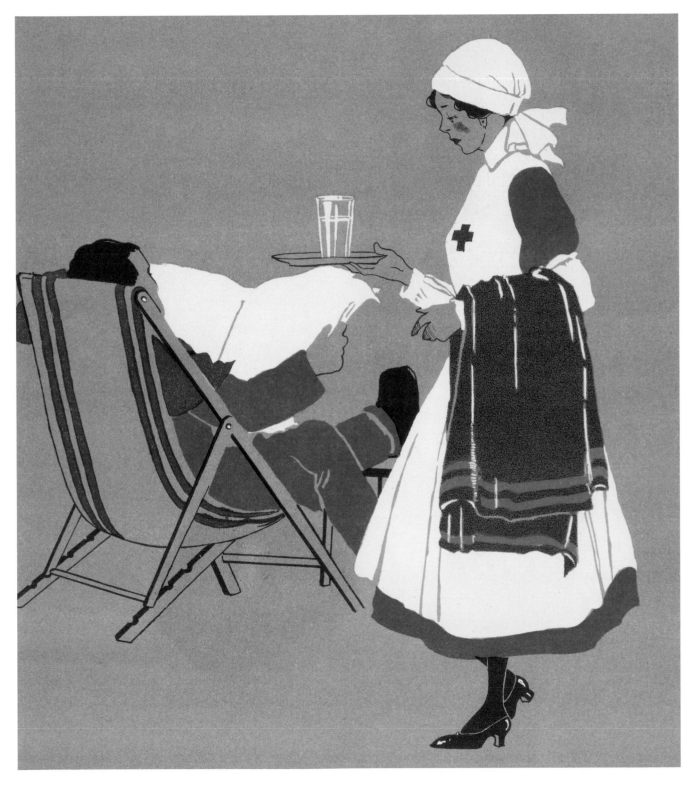

Index

Picture credits

The publishers would like to thank the following sources for their permission to reproduce the photographs and illustrations in this book:

Acknowledgments

The author would like to thank the following copyright holders for their kind permission to reproduce extracts:

The Hypatia Trust, Cornwall, for permission to reproduce an extract from: Violetta Thurstan, *Field Hospital and Flying Column: Being the Journal of an English Nursing Sister* (G. P. Putnam's Sons, London 1915)

Jurgen Wildner, for permission to reproduce an extract from a letter of Anna Fraentzel Celli.

Diggory Press, for permission to reproduce extracts from: Linda Richards, *America's First Trained Nurse* (Diggory Press, Liskeard, Cornwall, UK, 2006); Rosalind Franklin (ed.), *The Nightingale Sisters: The Making of a Nurse in 1800s America* (Diggory Press, Burgess Hill, West Sussex, UK, 2005)

The Jewish Women's Archive [http://jwa.org/exhibits/wov/wald/1w22.html], for permission to reproduce a verbatim quote of Lillian Wald.

Scribner, A Division of Simon and Schuster, Inc. for an extract from THE NATURE OF NURSING: A Definition and Its Implications for Practice, Research and Education by Virginia Henderson. Copyright © 1966 Virginia Henderson.

Every effort has been made to trace the copyright holders for the following texts, from which brief extracts have been taken:

Diack, Lesley, *Labrador Nurse* (Victor Gollancz Ltd, London 1963)

Gibbon, John Murray, *Three Centuries of Canadian Nursing* (The Macmillan Company, Toronto 1947)

Goodnow, Millie, *Outlines of Nursing History* (W. B. Saunders, Philadelphia 1923)

Luckes, Eva, *General Nursing*, Second Edition (Kegan Paul, Trench, Trubner and Co., London 1884)

McBryde, Brenda, *A Nurse's War* (Chatto and Windus, London 1979)

Nightingale, Florence, *Notes on Nursing* (Churchill Livingstone, London, 1980 edition)

Norris, Rachel, *Norris's Nursing Notes* (Sampson Low, Marston and Co., Ltd, London 1891)

Nutting, Adelaide, and Dock, Lavinia, *A History of Nursing: The Evolution of Nursing Systems from the Earliest Times to the Foundation of the First English and American Training Schools*, Four Volumes (G. P. Putnam's Sons, New York 1907/1912)

Sister Eva, *Scenes in the Life of a Nurse* (Bembrose and Sons, London 1890)

Stewart, Isla, and Cuff, Herbert E., *Practical Nursing*, Four Volumes (William Blackwood, Edinburgh 1899–1903).

We would be very grateful for any information that would enable us to trace these copyright holders.

The author would also like to acknowledge the generous help and support of Joan Lynaugh, Carol McCubbin (The Nurses' Voices Project'), Linda Shields, Pamela Wood, John and Susan Brocklehurst, Fiona Bourne (RCN Archives), Melissa Hardie (Hypatia Trust), Jonathan Evans (Royal London Hospital Archives), Suzanne Wingate, Felicia Cox, Patricia Davidson, Karen Clancy, Debbie Ciesielka, and Mary Ann Krisman-Scott. Also special thanks to Miren Lopategui for her patience, integrity, and commitment to this project.

Fil Rouge Press would like to thank:

Christine Hallett for her enthusiasm and authoritative research. Maura Buchanan for her support. Emily Hedges, Dave Jones, Miren Lopategui, and Kate MacPhee for all their hard work.

Nurses everywhere for their inspiring stories, courage, and caring.